GIRLS PLAY DEAD

JEN PERCY

GIRLS PLAY DEAD

Acts of Self-Preservation

Doubleday
New York

For my mother

I am convinced that during the Stone Age I must have been wounded by the love of some man, because a certain secret fear of mine dates from that time.

Be that as it may, one warm night, I was sitting and chatting politely with a civilized gentleman who was wearing a dark suit and had very correct fingernails. I was, as the writer Sérgio Porto would say, feeling perfectly at ease, and eating some guava. Then the man says: "Shall we go for a little ride?"

No. I'm going to tell the naked truth. What he said was: "Shall we go for a paseito*?"*

I didn't have time to find out the nature of that paseito, *because I immediately heard, coming from thousands of centuries, the rumble of the first stone in an avalanche: my heart. Who was it? Who, in the Stone Age, took me out for a* paseito *from which I never returned, because I'm still there?*

I don't know what hidden terror lies in the monstrous delicacy of that word paseito.

—CLARICE LISPECTOR, "In Favor of Fear"

... he kissed my eyes, and, mimicking the new bride newly wakened, I flung my arms around him, for on my seeming acquiescence depended my salvation.

—ANGELA CARTER, "The Bloody Chamber"

Author's Note

For the safety and privacy of some people I interviewed, I've occasionally used a pseudonym. While reporting on Debraca Harris, Antheshia Lee, and Laconda McDonald, I was granted access to the material in their resentencing petitions, and this material helped inform the women's stories.

GIRLS
PLAY
DEAD

Girl in the Snow

THERE IS NO SINGLE ANECDOTE. WHAT I'M TALKING ABOUT is an accumulation.

The man on the subway looks at my friend and me while he rubs his crotch. And we, not knowing how to react, stare ahead, waiting, ignoring it.

The man at the cash register begs me to let him touch my breasts before handing over my purchase: a bag of Skittles.

The gynecologist says, "Get undressed," but also says, "Keep the motorcycle boots on." I put my feet in the stirrups, boots on, and he caresses my thigh before he presses the speculum inside.

A man steals my purse and dangles it in front of me like a carrot all the way to his hotel room, where he sets it on the bed. He says that if I want my purse back, I have to come get it. I refuse to go in the room and so he dances with the purse and holds it like the body of a woman. He taunts me and I refuse again. But still I wonder, Am I ruining a good time?

Another man who wants to photograph me shows me the album of naked women. I'm sixteen. I remember how I say yes even though I'm thinking no. Not the word I'm hoping to say, not the word I'm thinking, anyway.

There's that professor with a gleaming head who starts

panting during class. Maybe a few of us are old enough to drink. He has his eyes closed, arms at his sides, while the panting and the moans—the *ohhs* and the *ahhs*—quicken. He screams and then his loose lips sputter like a balloon. "A female orgasm," he explains. He lifts a finger in the air, adjusts his blazer, and continues his lecture.

One summer after college, I rented a room in a house in Vermont with five men because the rent was cheap. At night when I came home from work, they would all be sitting together on the couch watching some sort of porn set in ancient Rome with gladiators and men who looked like Socrates. They always invited me to hang out. And I joined them because I didn't know what else to do. They were all really nice. They never touched me. There was just the porn, always on. I looked at the television and pretended to happily watch a man fuck a woman in a chariot while thinking about the nice girls who lived down the street in a clean house without porn, without the smell of old sex and old milk, with boyfriends who made love and parents who sent them on sailing trips for their birthdays.

There were times that I felt uncomfortable, or I didn't want to do what was being asked of me next. But I did. I went along with it, or I didn't say no, or I didn't leave, or I didn't want to be rude, or I thought I was overreacting, or I didn't want to hurt anyone's feelings, or I felt frozen and like I was no longer a part of the world. Times when I didn't make a fuss or whatever.

Here's the story of the Spanish man. I can still picture him—the Spaniard—eyes wet and black like those of a horse, wearing red swimming shorts and flip-flops thin as paper. I remember we were all in Seville and I was studying abroad. He was from the region, and we were all trying to meet locals to practice Spanish. He sat next to me and chewed a rolled cigarette. This was at a house party in a packed room where small blobs of slow-moving red light swam across the floor and up the walls. I was sitting on a couch and he sat down next to me. I turned to speak and he put his tongue in my mouth. When I pulled away, his bottom lip glistened. Behind us, shy girls crowded a snack table, spooning blue cake.

I remember the Spaniard and his friends were wearing fake mustaches. He tore off his mustache and handed it to me. In the glue, I spotted flakes of his skin. I put it on, and we laughed.

Later that evening, we walked together through the city's narrow streets, got lost in them. He showed me the best foods to order, the little snacks, the patatas and the shrimp and the pasta with squid ink. I had never been to Europe. He showed me the squares where everyone drank outside with ice in plastic cups.

He lived nearby and invited me over. We climbed the wooden stairs that spiraled in great wide turns to the top floor. The door to the apartment opened. It was a small apartment with tile floors. We ate sliced ham with melon. I noticed things: photos of saints, a figurine of a camel, ashtrays full of ash. I told him I wasn't going to have sex with him that night—that night in Seville. We kissed on the couch, and I said I should be going, but he pulled me closer. That's okay, he said, and he promised we wouldn't have sex. We kissed again. He said he wanted us to kiss naked. He wanted to hold me naked. I thought this sounded romantic. We undressed and were on the floor, and then he was going to put on a condom just in case. I thought of saying no one more time, but I was tired and I didn't want to be rude.

I also didn't want this to be something I *didn't* want.

Rape, I mean.

I kissed him back.

5

I wanted to see him again right away. I thought that by seeing him and spending time with him, it would mean we had spent a normal night together and this was a normal relationship. So the next day we explored the city, and I practiced Spanish. He asked me to travel with him to Paris—it was a work trip, but he invited me to come along. I had never been to Paris, and I told him all the things I wanted to do when we got there—visit the Café des Deux Moulins, walk along the Seine at night—and we did them. But mostly he left me alone to go work, and I wandered the city or stayed at home and watched the rain fall through the hotel windows. I remember a room so quiet I thought I could hear the flight of a passing bird.

There were always other cities, other work trips. We traveled to Amsterdam and Berlin, and smaller towns whose names I don't remember. When I told him I was worried about missing classes, he said things like "but you have me." So I stopped seeing friends and started skipping classes. At the same time, I didn't see much of him either: I was usually waiting for him to finish work, walking around, then going back to his hotel to have sex I did not enjoy.

I remember, on one of these trips, walking around Amsterdam one spring, when ice still formed on the streets. Everything smelled of fish and cold, the continuous thaw of earth. Snow arrived in quick bursts, falling infrequently but enough to be noticed and despised. The wooden walkway along the port was rotted by the North Sea. Women sat on benches facing the water, against cement walls, drinking out of flasks. Everywhere, pockets of steam lifted into the air. Nearby, a group of drunks were being evicted by the police. One man spun in a circle before he plummeted to the ground, arms spread like a snow angel.

I walked into a nameless bar where the ceiling fan wobbled

in a way that felt like another presence in the room. It had rained lightly, but there were cloud breaks in the sky, and it was that time of late afternoon when the light seemed orange instead of white and even a few insects were singing and active, moving along the windows. It was around when I often found myself alone, waiting for the Spaniard.

We didn't last long, just a few months. But there were times I didn't hear from him for a week. Two weeks. There were apologies, gifts.

"I loved you then," he'd say, "I will love you." As if to make me wait and wonder whether he loved me now. He said I had to be patient. I would be patient, I told him. I would wait.

I thought I was waiting for love. Waiting for warm hands, kind words, but I was also waiting to forget the things I didn't want—that night in Seville.

My friend offered me an anecdote stolen from a piece of writing by one of his students. In the story, there was a guy who texted a girl only when he wanted sex. Otherwise, he didn't talk to her. He ignored her on campus. One night it's snowing and below zero, and he tells her to come over. She is outside on the sidewalk. She says: Let me in. He tells her to wait because there's another girl there and he isn't sure what he wants—if he wants to be with her or not. He says he needs to think about it. He orders her to wait. The guy never texts again. The girl waits and waits. She doesn't have a coat, but she stays, waiting so long she doesn't notice that she is frozen—that she is dead.

There's a moment in Helen Garner's *The First Stone*: *Some Questions About Sex and Power* when Garner stops to try to remember her own "experience of being harassed by a man, the actual quality of the experience." A memory arrives—an incident from thirty years prior, when the author was on a train out of Melbourne. A man in his forties "who did not appear dangerous" sat beside Garner and started talking to her, all the while shifting his body closer to her own. They talked of horses and family. When the man put his arm around her shoulder, she didn't stop him. Next he asked Garner to give him a kiss. "I *let* him kiss me on the lips," she writes. But she wasn't sure if she allowed this "out of embarrassment, or politeness, or passivity, or a lack of a clear sense of what [*she*] wanted." There was no violence or force, Garner explains, no threat of any kind, just a steady persistence.

> What was my state, that allowed me to accept his unattractive advances without protest? I was just *putting up with him.* . . . I felt sorry for him. I went on putting up with him long past the point at which I should have told him to back off. *Should have?* Whose *should* is this? What I mean is *would have liked to. Wanted to but lacked the . . . the . . .* Lacked the what?

I earmarked the page and put it away. That was years ago, but I never forgot Garner's question. I, too, had done things I did not want to do. Mostly I was told I was passive or vulnerable, but it never felt that way to me.

Self-preservation doesn't always look like what we imagine it does. The woman who falls asleep next to her abuser isn't getting comfortable; she's experiencing the adrenaline dump that follows an experience of primal terror. The woman who lifts her hips to allow her attacker to take off her skirt is reverting to habits conditioned by years of sexism, racism, or abuse.

We learn that pleasing is the best way to react. That it's good to coax and be sweet. It's good to say, Do you want something? Can I help you? Do you want a massage? And sometimes we can avoid harm because we bring him some alcohol and he sleeps, and when he wakes we say, How are you?

We might start thinking about an abuser in a positive light; we might text to say: I had a good time last night, did you? Are you going to be at the party? I hope so! To say: You can't hurt me. Or we might fantasize about him, or spend more time around him, or have sex with him again, as if to say: Look, I'm fine.

A friend recommended I read "The Knife" by Joyce Carol Oates, and so I did. It's a short story about a mother, Harriet, who's at home with her young daughter when a robber appears. He doesn't find much to steal, so he points a knife at Harriet and tells her to get on the bed. Harriet tells the robber that she is afraid of the knife and begs him to put it down, and in response the robber lets her hold it.

And because she holds the knife, she wonders, "Is this rape?" And she wonders this even as the man pries "her legs apart" and pokes "himself against her."

Harriet reports the robbery, but not the rape, because she isn't sure how to explain the knife and why she didn't use it against her attacker.

A lawyer told me that most sexual assaults are not initiated by an attacker forcing somebody to acquiesce. So how are they able to do it? Why aren't we getting up and walking out? This was another question that troubled me. A question that contained my own passivity or, at least, accusations of passivity.

.   .   .

In Los Angeles, years ago, I was on my friend's bed with my legs folded to my chest, talking on the phone with my mom, when a man opened the door. He wore all black, with a gloved hand that held a knife. All the noise I'd been hearing in the kitchen wasn't my roommate, but this man. He must have thought no one was home. But this isn't about a robbery; it's about my reaction to it. I told my mom I had to go, and then I smiled at the man and said pleasantly, loudly, as gently as possible, *Hi.* The man ran off.

Why and when had I learned to respond to fear with a look of joy?

Bewilderment

Bewilderment (c. 1680) from Old English for "to take into the wilderness and get lost"

IN THE SUMMER, MY MOTHER AND I PRACTICED PLAYING DEAD in the woods. We practiced in the Three Sisters Wilderness, a volcanic part of the Cascade Range in central Oregon, where sunbaked pine perfumed the air. There were no grizzlies in Oregon, but we practiced anyway. My mother said I needed to practice because predators were less likely to eat dead things. She wore a safari hat and loose silky pants with leather hiking boots. She gave me the signal and I dropped to the ground, belly down, arms wide with my scabbed knees bent like a sprinter.

"Wrong," she said. "You look dead but it's not right."

My mother adjusted my death pose by tucking my legs under my belly and wrapping my arms over my neck like a scarf. Now I was a limbless thing with a backpack and a head. I looked like a turtle. She told me to hold steady. She told me to keep the pack on and let the bear paws tear it up. "This bear," she said, "prefers his prey alive."

My face was pressed into the dirt, sweet with the smell of ponderosa, the smell I associate most with childhood. Dirt, soft as flour, that settled on me like a second skin. I loved the smell. On hikes, I broke pine needles and wiped their wet centers on my skin like perfume. I could have easily been mistaken for a tree.

While I was death-feigning in the soft sweet dirt, my mother pretended to be a bear. She growled and snorted and pawed at my body to check for weakness. I closed my eyes and imagined her hands into paws. I imagined him on top of me. How could I trust myself to stay quiet beneath his wet sniffs? Those paws that did what they pleased. How long, really, could I wait?

I hated playing dead. I preferred to fight. I wanted to be loud and raise my pack high, shake my hands, and compete for wildness. I had done it before with a cougar on a trail in the Jefferson Wilderness.

"Wrong," she said again. "You look dead but it's not right."

I let my tongue hang limply from my mouth.

"Close," she said.

A final poke.

"Okay," my mother said. "You survived."

On weekends and in the summers, my mom and I drove into the wilderness. We drove with coolers packed with bags of Corn Nuts, Cool Ranch Doritos, processed pies topped with a shiny cinnamon glaze. We ate honey and peanut butter sandwiches. I was barely tall enough to see out the truck window. My hair was wild and fawn-colored. I wore shorts for climbing hills, and shirts with small animals on them. (My favorite had a big clownfish on it, the creature safe in a sea anemone's tentacles.)

We drove to wild places on thin roads that cut deep into the mountains until the asphalt gave way to dirt and the trees darkened the sky. We drove, and then we hiked, long hikes of ten or twenty miles, until we reached the soft light of the old-growth forests with their understories and nurse logs covered in tiny trees. We didn't see a lot of people, and people didn't see us. Just bears and shooting stars. I memorized the names of plants: red huckleberry and manzanita. Rhododendron, with its baby-pink flowers. Devil's club, with thorns on the underside of its leaves.

My mother had dark brown eyes and was bird-boned. She was a naturalist and the kind of woman who reached for keys in her pocket and came out with an owl pellet. Once I went into her wallet for a dollar and pulled out the skin of a small snake. I found a small pelvis bone in the sink. She collected pine cones, nests, leaves, and bones to bring home. I learned to do the same.

My earliest lessons on survival were from the animals and the trees. As we walked in the woods, she kept her eyes on the tops of the pines, because the bending and swaying of their crowns revealed to us how fast the wind was blowing and whether we needed to get home. Mapping the world for safety became second nature. Changes in elevation, the depth of sun, the length of shadow, the growth patterns of moss. She taught me to see the world as the animals did. How to lie low for a chipmunk's view; to look into dark places, into the foliage to catch sight of an ear or a predator's tail. I got used to spiderwebs in my mouth and gnats in my eyes.

I had a backpack with survival gear: a map, a peanut butter sandwich, a whistle, a space blanket, a matchbox, kindling, and water. We made time to practice surviving: I could hook a fish, build a shelter, read the stars.

We learned about the owl's silent flight, the porcupine's long defensive quills. About how the trees in danger could speak to each other with puffs of invisible chemicals or with their fungal roots that webbed the ground beneath us.

Moths grew wings with patterns like the faces of snakes or owls. Rabbits grew fur that changed with the seasons. Lizards could amputate their tails to get away.

I learned there were costs to self-preservation, that keeping ourselves safe meant we had to give something up.

I learned the horned lizard spurted blood from its eyes to scare predators. It made itself monstrous to stay alive. It gave up beauty.

The woods could be dangerous, but they were also a place of pleasure. We tried to feel everything our bodies could feel. We filled up on huckleberries, eating where the bears ate, right off the bush, fatting ourselves. I tasted bark, chewed bitter needles of pine and fir. Sweet pieces of hardened sap. The lemon pop of an ant. I put a moth wing in my mouth and it had a dusty taste.

I swam in glacial snowmelt that sucked blood from my extremities and made my lungs gasp for air. I let my toes bleed into mineral silt. I hiked on sprained ankles and broken bones. I figured out how to make my own splints. My ankle was always swollen—the ligaments torn and healing wrong. I learned to keep wounds a secret under my clothes and let them heal in the dark. I learned not to seek help for pain or to give a voice to wounds. After a plywood board at gym class tore into my shin, I went to the bathroom and stopped the blood with ropes of paper towel instead of using a Band-Aid. I pressed and patted the torn flesh back into my skin and it healed in lumps of scar tissue. I embraced my mother's stoicism. I even kept my period a secret and threw out the bloody clothes. My friends and I took turns wrapping our small hands on the electric horse fence to feel our hearts jump. It was a shock to the body, a submission to pain. We dared each other to do it in the rain.

. . .

If we weren't in the mountains to the west, then we were in the desert to the east. Almost half of Oregon is desert, all of it east of the Cascade Range, and it's an alien place. A visitor would find country covered in sagebrush and juniper, hills painted with belts of ochre, orange, brick-red sand, Mars-like pillars formed by waterfalls and volcanic sludge, volcanic uplifts, ancient seabeds, and between all this, small human settlements: wheat fields, alfalfa farms, cattle ranches.

Sometimes we brought the trailer, with its stale formaldehyde smell, lacquer table, and tiny fridge that gasped as if afraid. In the cabinets, a box of graham crackers, some marshmallows, and Hershey bars. Crystal Light powder that smelled both chalky and sour. Ketchup, mustard, relish.

Sometimes we slept on the ground in the valleys among the sagebrush in dust-coated sleeping bags beneath the thick porridge of the Milky Way. Sometimes we spent the night on the ground breathing volcanic ash with one ear pressed to the earth. We listened for geologic shifts, the belly of the earth settling. These sounds were the first sounds I spoke back to— the conversations I made with dust were the sounds of myself echoing back at me from the walls of volcanic rifts.

We visited caves, dead mouths of the earth, cold and low on oxygen. We threw headlamp beams at the walls.

Days passed without the sight of another human. I was scabby and bleeding and coated in dust.

One summer day I waited for my mother in a field of lupine. It was her favorite flower, tall and fluffy like lavender ice cream. She was slower than me on hikes, so I usually walked ahead and then waited for her to catch up. When she arrived, thirty minutes later, we ate honey sandwiches. Birds circled the sky.

That was when I asked my mother about her pain, because she had been limping on the trails, stopping often to rest. She was always trying to hide the pain, and I often found her at home in bed with the lights off, chewing pills in a neck brace.

She told me about the day she almost died in the woods, and how it began with crotch shots. "The walls were covered in crotch shots," she said. She was talking about the walls of the office at the scaling yard outside Crow, Oregon, the walls plastered with pages torn out of *Playboy* or *Penthouse*. She was twenty-two. This was her first job out of college; the first that wasn't babysitting or refilling water glasses at the diner. She didn't love the logging industry—in fact she hated it—and she wanted to make it better. This job was a place to start, a place to get dirt under her nails, the sun in her hair, and a line on her résumé. While looking at the crotch shots, she remembered the apartment where she lived with my dad in the city, and the man who always cornered her in the hall when she was alone, chasing her while chanting *I want to lick your pussy, I want to lick your pussy.*

The men—her colleagues—were looking at her looking at crotch shots, so she turned away from them, sat down, and just chatted about work.

She came every day when they told her to come. She carried a clipboard and tape, a hard hat and a vest. She wore plaid shirts and jeans. Her hair was long, dark, and parted at the center. Everyone called her "girl." She was five foot three but not a girl.

All men, all around. She tried to focus instead on how lucky she was to be out in the wilderness, where she had always wanted to be ever since her father brought her out of the city for the first time to see a turquoise river called the Metolius. She remembered touching the cold water until her fingers turned red as if burned.

But the men at the scaling yard wanted her to leave, and they let her know it. You're the kind of woman who steals jobs from men, they told her.

A month passed before my mother's supervisor—a big man, she remembered, with a red goatee, a Paul Bunyan tattoo, and a missing finger—pulled her aside and told her that he was sorry, but she would need to leave.

My mother asked why. He shifted his weight and folded his arms. He told her it was because of the way she was bending over when she was measuring the logs. He accused her of "being distracting" and that she was "liable to cause an accident" because the men were looking at her ass.

He called her inappropriate for the way she moved and dressed and spoke.

"It was like everything was my fault," my mother told me.

They transferred her to a different job in another wilderness area, bright with towering Douglas fir, a place she would be hidden from these men. The new job had her going into clear-cuts to measure regrowth. One day her supervisor, a young guy in Carhartt jeans and matching jacket, asked her to survey trees on an area of land near a cliff. Mom leaned forward to get a better view of the cliff's edge, sparsely covered in Douglas fir, bordered by aster and wild huckleberry. The area he wanted surveyed was covered by an eroded rockfall called scree. It could be dangerous, slippery as ice.

She didn't want to lose her job or cause more trouble, because she already felt like she was causing trouble. But she told him anyway how she didn't think it was safe. He ignored her plea and told her to finish her job.

"It was like his voice was moving me," my mother explained. "Pushing me forward. I had abandoned my own thoughts."

All around, tiny trees pushed their way up through the

rocks. She found one sapling, and then another. Trees with trunks flimsy as licorice sticks.

When the scree gave way, knocking over my mother, she somersaulted several hundred feet down to the cliff's edge. All that saved her was a sapling she snatched. The roots held her weight.

Her hand was bloodied. The bark tore her skin. A bruise canvased her body, from her knees clear past her hip bone. It looked like a continent, like her body was a map. Her supervisor carried her to the truck and drove her home. On the drive, pain had her going in and out of consciousness, but she refused to go to the hospital.

She didn't want her supervisor to get in trouble, she told me. It was all she thought about.

That same week a clot formed in my mother's arteries and she had a stroke that left her nearly blind in one eye. And because of where the bruise was located, near her pelvis, near her womb, she had paranoid thoughts about whether she would be able to have children.

"Things would be different now," she told me. "Now I would report it. But at the time, well, it was like I gave him my power."

I try to remember the first time I gave up my power, the first submission.

My mother was in the kitchen washing vegetables when the phone rang.

She wiped her hands on her skirt to answer. "Yes," she said, and then "wait a minute." She covered the phone and whispered, "It's for you."

I was sitting at the kitchen table eating an after-school

snack. I pressed my nails into the wood and scratched. I wasn't expecting anyone. I walked down the hall and took the phone.

"Hey, baby," the voice said. "It's me. It's Sean, baby."

I didn't know any Seans. He sounded old.

"Hi," I said.

I thought I should tell Sean that we'd never met, but I didn't.

My mom stared right at me. I pressed the phone to my ear and tilted my head like I was interested. She looked away.

"This is you, Jenny, right?"

"Yeah," I said.

"Are you tired? What's wrong?"

"I dunno," I said. "I'm fine. I'm just sick."

"I miss you," he said. "I love you."

"I love you too," I whispered.

I hung up the phone and went back to my snacks. Milk and Oreos. When my mom asked who it was, I said some kid at school.

That night, I pulled my polyester rainbow comforter up to my chin and thought about Sean. He'd have freckles, I imagined, and hair like a dust mote. He'd be sweat-stained and know how to drive a tractor. He'd have a way with horses.

Sean called again. I talked to him like I was his girlfriend the best I could. I liked saying I love you. *I love you too.*

When we talked again, I remember his voice changed to something low and quick. "I want you. I want you right now. I want to fill you with my cum until there's nothing else left of you."

I said nothing. I had no idea what he was talking about.

"What's wrong?" he said.

"I can't be all cum," I said and hung up.

. . .

For many years my parents lived off the land outside Eugene, Oregon, tilling the earth, planting crops. My father brought home animals, dragged elk out of the woods and let the blood drain in the garage. He wore blaze orange on a hunt, and when he returned home, there was always pinesap still soft in his beard, a few leaves stuck to his shoulder, and sometimes he was dragging a four-prong buck behind him like a bag of laundry. I remember him explaining that there were two ways to hang a deer: from its neck or from its legs. He preferred the neck. I watched from inside our kitchen—windows open, screens shut—as my father worked the knife through a tough spot on the deer's stomach. It hung from an old juniper tree, its neck twisted ninety degrees. My father made an incision and peeled the skin off leisurely and with care, the way he might take off a woman's jacket at a party. It made a sound. He turned, he explained: The sooner you skin the deer after it dies, the easier the hide slides off. The deer was naked, purple and soft, like the deepest part of a peach.

Once, I joined my father on an elk hunt. We waited on a logging road that overlooked a meadow. There were purple flowers in the meadow and a small stream, and parts were heavy with mist. When the elk arrived with their soft smoky chests, I screamed to save them. My father lowered his rifle, packed the car, and we drove home. We never spoke of this.

But I was fed the elk—the ones he killed.

After my mother's job with the Forest Service, after the accident, she didn't find another job in the woods, but worked at a restaurant called Mr. K's in the Bend River Mall where for eight hours every day she counted grease-stained receipts and watched employees flip T-bone steaks and pull little hairs out of the coleslaw salad. Mr. K's was full of green vinyl booths and pink-framed Monet posters, synthetic flowers that smelled like cigarettes, and pies that incubated for days under the fluorescent lights of a plastic display case. My father had a mustache. My mother put in curlers every morning. I had to go to the mall, too, and it wasn't one of those malls with loud music and rides and people getting makeovers and old ladies doing their morning workouts, but one of those malls where you can see from one side to the other and the ceiling is low and dim and the color of dishwater.

When my mother met my father in high school, she spent evenings and weekends at his house. By the time she turned eighteen, they were married and living on their own. When she married my father, it was for the reasons a lot of women marry: for love, and to escape.

My mother was raised in Portland by Nana, my grandmother, whom my mom described as a "lunatic." Nana had round sunken eyes, thick gold-framed glasses, and a poodle perm. She was four foot eight and every year she grew smaller. Her house smelled like ripe fruit and rodents. Nana's uniform consisted of a purple tracksuit and white sneakers—we could always hear the swoosh and crackle of her approach. She squealed when she saw me. She said a ghost lived in her basement, but we were not allowed to talk about *him*. We lived on one side of the Cascades and she lived on the other—the wilderness was a boundary between us. When we saw Nana— almost always for Christmas or Thanksgiving—we drove over the mountains, often in deep, blinding snow.

My mother remembered how Nana punished her with chores, making her get down on her knees to scrub vinyl floors, swirling a blue chemical spray on windows until the rag squeaked, until her clothes dampened with cleaning solvents and the pads of her fingers turned smooth. Nana checked for smudges, and if the house wasn't clean enough she'd tell my mom to start again. My mother was the only girl of Nana's four children and it was just assumed that cleaning was her job. Every night, my mother cooked dinner and cleaned up after everyone else. She remembered her brothers did nothing and were asked to do nothing. They lounged by the television while she scrubbed away. She hardly had time to study. My mother was also always sickly, often plagued by pneumonia. One year she missed fifty days of school, and her teachers stopped by for welfare checks. She spent weeks in the hospital alone—Nana never visited.

When I talked to my mother about Nana, it was a story of neglect. It was a story of being without a mother. In fact, Nana was devoted to another mother—Elizabeth Clare Prophet—the leader of the Church Universal and Triumphant, which began in Los Angeles and ended in Bozeman, Montana. Prophet was known to her spiritual followers as the Mother. And Mother is exactly how Nana expected to be addressed by her children, who were always asking, Where is Mother? Or, Why is Mother standing on her head?

The day Nana left for the cult, my mother found her in the kitchen wrapping brownies in tinfoil. Nana dragged suitcases into the garage and packed the car. She said she was leaving for a long time.

"Do you really want to be around if everyone else is dead?" my mother asked.

"Oh yes," Nana said. "We are the destined."

Elizabeth Prophet was a New Age guru with the same poodle cut as Nana. She had inherited the church in 1973 after the death of her husband, Mark Prophet. Under her leadership the number of followers grew from hundreds to thousands. Congregations spread across the globe, and she published more than fifty books about the group. She was not a feminist but rewrote the church's theology to appear to give more power to women. She liberated both sexes from the guilt of original sin, referred to God as both Father and Mother, brought messages from female beings like the Virgin Mary and the Hindu goddess Durga. She claimed gender had no bearing on how far anyone could climb up the spiritual ladder.

Nana left that night and moved onto 12,500 acres of land on the border of Yellowstone National Park. She prepared to go underground to survive. Members bought radiation suits, ordered ammunition in military calibers, cleared local stores of camping and survival gear. The bunkers were 20 feet deep and, together, big enough to house 750 people. They had kitchens, showers, laundry, an infirmary. Cult members installed seat belts on the bunk beds. Followers donated their savings and worked for free. During this time, Prophet got pregnant with the Messiah and then miscarried.

The end of the world was set for March 15, 1990. This was during the Cold War, and Prophet thought the Russians were going to nuke the Pacific Northwest. She'd been eavesdropping on Mikhail Gorbachev by "mind traveling" to the Kremlin. It's how she knew about the nukes and how she knew fluoride was a Russian plot to gain control over the Americans. If the nukes didn't kill everyone, she explained, something else would. The end of the world meant they'd be free to start a new civilization. Most of the members were women. And these were women who looked forward to the end of the world. "A golden age," Elizabeth Prophet's daughter wrote in her memoir about the cult, the one that was coming after the apocalypse, "is what the older ladies in our church had been hoping for since the 1930s." Maybe the women would wake up and they'd be in charge?

My mother recounted the story to me in horror, uttering over and over, "I can't believe we're related! If I ever end up like Nana, kill me!"

But the more I understood about Nana's childhood, the more I understood her decision to join a cult. There weren't many decisions to be had. Nana was raised by an abusive father in destitution. She had a cousin named Betty who lived with Nana. They were raised like sisters. I remember Betty, a chain-smoker on a musty floral couch, eating expired candy from a cut glass bowl. It was Betty who told us this story about Nana's parents: how her mother took a kitchen knife and stabbed Nana's father in the heart. She had watched the stabbing from the living room and remembered the blood on his hands. He'd refused to go to the hospital because he didn't want anyone to ask questions. He didn't want the violence to be known. They decided that he "slipped and fell on the knife."

When my mother was sixteen, she went to visit Betty's husband. Mom told me how he assaulted her and tried to take off her clothes. How he ran his hands up and down her body, all over her breasts, between her legs. "I couldn't move," she told me. "It was very confusing." It lasted a couple minutes and then she sprinted out the door, drove back to Nana's house, locked the door, sat on the couch. She was home alone. Then she saw a shadow behind the little window on the front door. He had followed her. He banged and rattled. She hid in the bathroom with the door locked, and she curled into herself. It was as deep and safe as she could get. She sat there hoping he wouldn't get in. That his shadow wouldn't darken the light under the door.

.   .   .

I knew about Nana's cult before I knew about my mother's guru. Her name was Ida Rose Barber, and she attracted a lot of West Coast hippies whom she hypnotized on her couch. (The poet Allen Ginsberg had asked her for help with his paralyzed face.) "A small woman," my mother remembered, "incredibly small, with long white hair, who spoke a thousand miles an hour. The most frightening woman." Ida Rose hypnotized my mother for years. She put my mother into trance states and took notes while my mother babbled words and conjured stories. Hypnosis and trance released her from her own body. Eyelids fluttering, going elsewhere, better than here.

While my mother was in a trance, Ida Rose told her things about herself—who she was and what she wanted. She told her about her "past lives." My mother was able to imagine inhabiting other bodies, usually of men, or powerful women, never ordinary ones. In one life, she's a woman in Scotland who cuts off her braids and disguises herself as a man so she can fight a war. In another, she's a heroic woman freeing persecuted Christians from prison. In yet another, she's a pioneer shooting at bandits with a rifle.

"When I woke up from the trance," my mother said, "I felt known for the first time."

One day my mother mailed me a manila envelope with copies of the past-life readings. I was surprised they existed, but Ida Rose's followers always transcribed the readings with a typewriter and my mother had kept all the copies. I was reading these transcriptions when I learned Ida Rose put her hands on my mother's pregnant stomach and gave a reading of my unborn self. (I was from the time of Charlemagne, something about the pope regalia.) These were stories about me before I was born, still growing in the womb. One story was dark and worrisome. It was about my mother's injury after her fall, and how the pregnancy was hurting her back and might eventually kill her. The reading—which was also a kind of prophecy—said I was going to be born a boy, but because I was hurting my mother, I flipped over in the womb and transformed into a girl. The transcription read: It would rather come in masculine, but it was concerned for the mother. So it was thinking maybe it should come in feminine.

I liked the fact that in this story I was being kind to my mother and easing her pain, but I didn't like that it had to do with me being a girl. It was a story that defined me before I had a chance to define myself, before I could open my mouth and speak. A script shaping a girl. A girl who accommodated the pain of others. I never thought it could start so early.

When I was sixteen, my mother and I were in our truck driving somewhere when she told me a story about "these men bothering her" at a trailhead, looking at her, getting close. When she got in her truck, they got in their own. They followed her when she circled the lot. "I feel like I just attract these men," she told me. We were quiet. "It must have had something to do with one of my past lives," she added. I rolled my eyes and looked out the window at the passing trees.

My mother's stories were sometimes infused with the spiritual: miracles, ghosts, and prophecy. "Don't deny your talents," my mother told me. You feel things, she said, you see things. Do you feel the ghost? Is it here? I remember wanting this to be true and also hating that it could be true. I was a fearful child and very afraid of the dark. At night, I found my hands clasped in prayer, asking for safety, but otherwise didn't feel drawn to belief. Not in the sunlight, not in the daylight.

In the nineteenth century, women used the supernatural as a path to power, and channeling the voices of the dead was one of the few career opportunities available to women.

It gave them a chance to inhabit forbidden male roles— to travel and have sexual adventures. Often these were poor women of low social standing. Almost all felt they didn't have power until they channeled the voices of the dead. Nettie Colburn Maynard was a young and illiterate woman from upstate New York, but served as a medium for Abraham Lincoln's wife, and in a trance, she would communicate with spirits then offer advice to White House officials. Maynard wrote in her diaries that officials "lost sight of the timid girl . . . and seemed to realize that some masculine spirit force was giving speech to almost divine commands."

The historian R. Laurence Moore wrote that many women were "seized" by male spirits and spoke in the voices of men, including "swearing sailors, strong Indian braves, or oversexed male suitors." In one séance, Moore writes, a female medium channeled a "firm, erect military man." Channeling the dead also helped many nineteenth-century women divorce their husbands, because a male spirit granted them permission.

It was a path to power but also a giving up of the self— whether to male spirits or a cult leader. The individual was abandoned for the group. What felt like freedom was also a kind of capture.

My mother and I never talked about our fears, but we sometimes talked about our dreams. We dreamed of predation. She dreamed of cougars, who came to her as she slept, quiet in the tomb of night. Once, she woke up with her hands around her neck, and she was choking herself because she thought the cougar was ripping out her throat. I dreamed of a shark. I was with him in the ocean at dusk, just me and him. Sometimes he slipped into my daydreams. There was a lot of fear, a lot of anxiety, but always unarticulated—always suspended in the symbolic.

One day my mom turned to me and said, "Did I tell you about the raccoon blood?" That morning, she went to the backyard and discovered blood in the birdbath. The railing was also covered in an enormous amount of blood. She spent a long time looking for the raccoon by following his bloody prints. The afternoon rain didn't wash away the blood, so she had to start scrubbing it off with a sponge. "They have human hands," she said, "with long fingers. The shape of a rainbow."

I asked if she could show me the prints and she shook her head. Outside, the sun was low. She refused to go out at dusk. "It's their time," she said. Meaning the animals.

When I was fourteen years old, Mom and I were at a stoplight in a construction zone on a country highway. The sun was bright and it was hot. Mom chewed on some Corn Nuts and looked at the intersection's yellow blinking streetlight wobbling in a warm gust of wind. Men worked the ground, making holes in the earth, piling dirt. My mother and I were quiet.

"All these men," she said. "All of these men are looking at you." I was too young for this. They were not looking, not at all.

I remember when my father showed us his gun. We found him standing silently in the living room, his body contorted into an elegant pose, gun tilted up toward the ceiling. It was a 9mm semiautomatic with a tactical beam light and laser sight with a seventeen-round magazine. He demonstrated the laser feature by drawing shapes on our foreheads. We just stared and asked if it was loaded, but my mother assured us. Dad would never bring a loaded gun in the house, she said. She wore an apron covered in flour and pressed pie dough into a pan.

"My mother was born into this," I told a friend.

"But so were you," she said. "Weren't you also born into this?"

When I was in high school, we moved to Portland and lived in a cheap apartment. (We moved five times in those four years, all within the city.) The first place was one of those apartments among hundreds of apartments that all look the same. It was behind a grocery store called Fred Meyer, where the dumpsters filled with stale birthday cake. I remember the sky was a perpetual gray and the rain fell in long swipes.

My mother was in her bedroom lying on the bed in the dark. My father was somewhere on a business trip. I could tell she was sad being away from the woods.

When a senior from another school started calling in the evening, I thought it was a chance to make a friend. We met at a soccer match, or at a party, I don't remember. "What do your nipples look like?" he said when he called. He gave me a list of coins I could use to describe my nipples. "Are they quarters?" he asked me. "Are they nickels?" He offered colors: petal pink to coffee brown.

I didn't really know what was normal and what wasn't. He called night after night, getting more and more of me.

One day the senior and I got high using a Pepsi can. He went first and passed me the can, and I put my lips where his lips had been and it felt like a first kiss without actually kissing.

When he invited me to a party, I said yes. It was a crowded party in a basement with a rusty fridge stocked with Budweiser and salami. The light was a thick purple down there, and people moved in and out of the basement as if emerging from a pool. I opened the fridge and a square of light framed my body.

The carpet was soft and so were the chairs. In a sliding glass door, our reflections moved about brightly as if on a screen. In the corner of the room, someone slept in a beanbag chair. I drank enough to be tired, and I was on the floor waiting for the senior and listening to the music when someone crawled on top of me. I thought it was the senior. I was happy to see him. I held him and kissed his shoulders. But instead I found myself looking into the eyes of a strange man. I stiffened. He touched me and rubbed my breasts. His weight made it hard to breathe. I felt light, floating, no longer afraid. I heard the sound of the ocean.

He crawled away. "Sorry," he said.

I sat up. There were vacuum tracks on the carpet and family photographs on the wall.

I was thinking of how strange I felt, like my body had left me, and that I had been warm and closer to God than I had ever been. I was becoming spiritual like my mother and my grandmother, I thought. I didn't want to be this way, and I wondered if I should tell my mother. But I knew what she would say—that I had special powers and needed to use them.

In the kitchen, on my way out, a girl brushed my sweater. "I saw you," she said. She looked to be sixteen, the same age as me. "Looked like you had fun," she said. I turned around to see where she was pointing. She was pointing at him: the strange man in the dark. The party had spread to the living room, where he broke into a wild, butt-shaking dance, moving low to the floor and waddling with his arms flapping like a duck.

She thought that I wanted it. Did I? I reacted as if I did. It was too difficult to explain, I told her. I shrugged and left.

———

I thought little of the creepy man in the dark. I only thought: I am strange. I didn't know what my body did when it was afraid. I spent years living in the world not understanding the behaviors that rose up suddenly during or after fear. What did fear even look like? How do you tell stories about it? Maybe after so much time in the woods dreaming of survival, I became too confident in my imagination of what I could do to keep safe. My mother thought she could keep me safe from bears, which would translate to keeping me safe from men.

What made Helen Garner recoil, finally, away from the man on the train? "What stopped it," she wrote, "was that somebody walked past the compartment and looked in. Suddenly I saw through that unknown witness's eyes what was happening to me, what I was failing to object to. I saw that it was absurd. And I slid out of his grip and left the compartment."

It was as if she had been held by the strange man's vision of the world, and then, all at once, escaped back into her own. It made sense—men had been controlling this script for so long that she was engulfed by his vision of normalcy. A stranger caused a fissure, a disruption.

Sometimes the stories of strangers in books serve this purpose too. They can help us feel less alone, less strange. So I started collecting these stories.

I remembered that in *A Girl's Story,* the author had offered the man who violated her some hazelnut chocolate milk from her parents' store. So I asked, as a beginning, What normalizing thing did you do immediately after your rape?

I comforted him and said it was okay. I told him I was totally fine.

I convinced him to be my boyfriend and then we went to a movie.

I comforted him because he was crying.

I made him chicken soup. I brought him a blanket. I spent the night looking out the kitchen window in silence.

I acted like he was the victim and I told him I was sorry.

We talked about our future together. All the trips we would take.

I had a bath and watched television with my family.

I fell asleep next to him.

I took a nap with him.

I cuddled him.

I went to church.

I told him I couldn't wait to do it again.

What I Look Like When I'm Afraid

MY FRIENDS AND I WENT SWIMMING IN LAKES IN THE SUMmers. Different friends, different lakes. I remember summer camp at a lake rimmed with pine, eating licorice whips and drinking Diet Coke, reading too many copies of *Cosmopolitan* magazine, taking quizzes (are you more of a lion or a rabbit?) while running oil up our legs. And I remember how one of these summers I wouldn't swim. I just walked the edges of the shore. I turned to look at the lifeguard, but he was not looking, he was sitting alone on a rock, staring at something in the lake. But I thought about him looking at me.

When anyone asked why I didn't swim, I said "because I'm not a good swimmer" or "I don't feel like it." I sat on the shore and let the water lap at my feet. I wiped the dirt caught between my toes. I was thinking more about what my body would look like drowning. I would look ugly, I thought. I would make embarassing sounds and I would make the lifeguard think of a wet cat; I wouldn't have control of my body. At thirteen, the thought of this was much worse than drowning.

My grandmother Louise—not my cult grandma, but my other one—was a nervous woman who suffered from panic attacks and didn't leave the house for long periods. She grew so pale that her skin almost brightened from the absence of sun, became like a slab of marble. Over the years, it turned a bit feathery from all the powder she used, and it reminded me more and more of the skin of brie than anything of flesh or stone. She lived in a small house in Salem, Oregon, and styled herself as a middle-class Marie Antoinette with fake gold-rimmed mirrors, crystal chandeliers, velvet couches, and a finely primped toy poodle. She threw tea parties for her teddy bears and tended a garden with a cherub fountain. Every doorknob had a tassel.

There were two places this Louise would go. To the store that sold tassels or to the local pancake house. She always arrived like a hostage, with watery eyes. It was agony. If she needed to use the bathroom, she would have to wait. She could not pass through a crowd.

I remember being at a grocery store with her one time, and we were waiting in line when, suddenly, she stilled. A cantaloupe was in her hand, scratchy and cool, and I saw that her thumb sank into a wet crater of blue and white mold. There was a pungent, sweet odor.

I saw her staring at the pile of cantaloupes near the entrance and I imagined she wished to go get another, but she could not do it. She glanced at the line of people behind her, and I saw a slight tremor in her hand. She must have seen what looked like a centipede of human eyes glittering above shopping carts. She continued on, setting the melon down to ride the belt.

William James in 1890 considered "the strange symptom" of agoraphobia a survival strategy that humans had evolved away from but that was chronic in wild animals and domestic cats who only ventured out into the open "as a desperate measure." To James, the agoraphobic reverts to an animal state, a state of being prey, and experiences "terror at the sight of any open place or broad street which he has to cross alone."

The agoraphobic ones lose sleep, hyperventilate, and cry at the thought of going into public. It means they can't step outside to empty the trash, get the mail, buy groceries. Heavy blinds and blackout curtains are important, and so are locks. Some have to hype themselves up for weeks or months in advance. They try to do fun things near their door to build positive associations with the outside. Maybe they move past the front door to the front steps, then to the driveway and to the mailbox.

Ann Seagrave and Faison Covington were agoraphobic psychologists who coauthored *Free from Fears: New Help for Anxiety, Panic and Agoraphobia.* Covington mistook her first panic attack for a stroke because she was seeing black spots and couldn't feel her arms. Seagrave had her first attack driving down an unfamiliar road when her "body went berserk" and "a host of other horrifying sensations began to surface." She became hot and sweaty, although she was shaking as if cold. Her vision blurred and her feet went so numb that she didn't believe she could brake the moving car. "Our bodies act in a way that is, for us, terrifying," Seagrave wrote.

Psychologists talk about panic attacks as "catastrophic misinterpretations" of normal sensations of anxiety. Palpitations, breathlessness, dizziness are thought to be evidence of a heart attack, a brain hemorrhage, a slip into insanity.

A nineteenth-century doctor named Carl Westphal chose the word "agora," the ancient Greek for marketplace or a public place of assembly. Agoraphobia, then, is a "fear of public places." Westphal, however, did not think patients feared public places but, rather, feared the panic they felt in those places. It wasn't open spaces, but peopled ones. It's "the fear of fear." And the fear of panic itself develops over time into agoraphobia.

Things agoraphobics fear: that someone could talk to you, or that someone could look at you in a weird way. That you might have to make a quick decision, or that you might faint. Maybe that someone will notice you're anxious and will try to help you, and you might not know how to answer a stranger's question. Or maybe you'll have a heart attack and the paramedics will expose your breasts. They worry about the staring, the hovering, the questions from strangers.

Men are almost as likely as women to suffer from panic attacks, but women with panic attacks are more likely to develop agoraphobia. There are simply more consequences for women looking "out of control" in public. They worry that if they have a panic attack, people will see a deviant or misbehaving woman. They picture their own psychic and bodily sensations of panic but also what they believe other people see.

When I asked friends and strangers about what they imagined when they thought of an "out of control" body, some said things like screaming, convulsing, or throwing plates at a window, but many said more ordinary things: urinating, fainting, vomiting, laughing, blushing, sweating, loud breathing, stomach grumbling, farting, burping. In other words, to be "out of control" was simply to be a body in the world. One little gurgle could cause a spiral.

When geographer Ruth Bankey interviewed agoraphobic women in Scotland, she found that they often assumed others could see what they were feeling internally, though so often their experiences of panic weren't visible at all. (Perhaps there were cues like pale skin, sweat, quick short breaths.) Catherine, a woman in her mid-forties, worried people could see that she was "losing control" of her body, and that other people would see her as "unreal," "fading away," and "screaming." Lisa, a teenager, reported "people would see a woman, me, collapse, big dramatic crash." Bankey calls this a fear of the hysterical image—"a fear of being perceived by others as excessively feminine, out of control, and slipping into madness . . . that one's experiences will not be taken seriously."

———

Sarah is a twenty-six-year-old agoraphobic sex worker who hasn't left her apartment for two years because she is afraid of floating into the sky. At home, her style leans sexy Victorian goth—black hair, red lips, pale skin. She lives in a one-bedroom apartment in Omaha—a big complex next to a gas station and a Hy-Vee. The worn carpet is beige and the walls are white. A sliding glass door gives her access to a patio where wolf spiders spook her in the morning.

The days are not hard to fill. It is not as boring as one might think. She checks her email and social media, and then plays "brain training" games online so she doesn't get dementia, which is one of her major worries. Then she does "exposure therapy" by standing on the patio beneath the sky. "The sky terrifies me," she said. "It's so big and vast." Every day, she paces around the apartment for thirty minutes until she starts to sweat. That is her exercise.

In the beginning, she made it a goal to walk to the church across the street and get some pamphlets, maybe even start going to mass. She made it to the parking lot and then turned around and ran home.

Sometimes she walks in the grass just outside the apartment. She especially likes it when it snows. She even brought one of her cats outside for a walk on his birthday, but he didn't like the snow on his paws. She has an orange cat and a black cat and spends a lot of time with them. "Dennis and Dexter, my little serial killers," she says. "I would die without them."

Sarah told me she had never experienced the warmth of another person. Never had a relationship that was safe. She was a middle schooler in Michigan when her life got derailed by an older girl named Savannah.

"Basically, she would give me drugs, get me high, tell me to have sex with guys, and buy me something nice," she told me. Savannah collected money from the guys. It was trafficking, but Sarah didn't know that's what was happening.

Savannah groomed Sarah for a year before pimping her out. "Savannah knew it would be easy with me," Sarah explained. Because she was bullied a lot in middle school and high school, she kept to herself. "I was fat," Sarah explained, "that was a big one. I was poor and didn't have name-brand clothes, and I smelled of cigarettes because my mom smoked like a chimney. Well, and I was bullied because I was gay." Savannah zeroed in on her because she liked to find victims who no one would notice disappear. "Which, in my case," Sarah told me, "was true."

When Sarah was seventeen, she complained to a guy on a dating site about Savannah. Early on, she pressured Sarah to lose her virginity when she invited her to some house party, pointed to a guy, and said, "I know he will sleep with you." The guy got drunk and Sarah got buzzed. They went back to a bedroom, had sex, and left blood on the bed. After somebody found the blood, they were checking all the girls' panties for it.

Sarah said Savannah had done it to other girls. There was one right after Sarah who she trafficked in Florida. That girl had a trick baby and killed herself.

The man on the dating site was twenty-five, and Sarah thought she was in love with him. He told her, "If you come to Texas, I won't do that to you." So she went to Texas and ended up right back in the same situation. He took her to a hotel and she started making a few hundred dollars a day.

"I loved him so much," she told me. "I was already conditioned to believe that if you love somebody, you do that for them. I didn't know what a healthy relationship looked like." She was jailed for prostitution, still not understanding that it was trafficking. She turned eighteen in rehab, went to a transitional living facility, relapsed, and went right back to the streets.

She did sex work in Wisconsin, Florida, Illinois, and Michigan. It was all she knew how to do to keep herself fed and alive. She was abandoned at truck stops and slept at children's shelters. She kept Mace strapped to her wrist with a rubber band, hid a knife in her garter, and put sharp bobby pins in her hair. One night in a Walmart parking lot a customer tried to rape her and she stabbed his eye with a bobby pin. Another time a customer strangled her with an extension cord, and she wiggled away just enough to shoot Mace between them. He stumbled out the door and she pushed him over the motel balcony. He fell two stories onto asphalt but sprung up like a cat and ran off.

Before the apartment in Omaha, she lived in a van for almost two years, sleeping at Walmart or hospital parking lots. And before the van, she lived in a house with several men who covered expenses in exchange for sex. When the pandemic arrived, they kicked her out. She bought a 2006 Ford and pushed a mattress inside. She drove through Oklahoma, Florida, Georgia, Alabama, Mississippi, and Texas. She spent the spring in Nebraska. Summertime she went north to Wisconsin, Michigan, and Minnesota. She never felt safe. While parked at an abandoned mall in Georgia, she woke up to find a man with a crowbar trying to open the driver's door. She was naked and thought: He's going to rape me. She made sure to put on a T-shirt before she slipped into the driver's seat and started the engine. The agoraphobia began around this time. She noticed she was always worrying about dying. It started on a bridge, she remembered. Would the bridge collapse? She wasn't sure, so she stopped driving on bridges. I'm going to die in the heat, she thought, or I'm going to freeze in the cold. Or my van is going to roll away into the lake, or into a tree. She wondered if a tree would fall and crush the van in her sleep. She stopped driving on the interstate. She stopped eating outside. At night, she often opened her eyes to look at the driver's seat because maybe a man was there driving her into the night. That's when the sky grew ominous. That's when she felt like she wasn't real anymore, and that the boundaries of her body were not enough to keep herself safe. She didn't understand what was happening. "I thought it was something spiritual," she told me. "That I was going through a spiritual experience." She didn't know she was having panic attacks until she listened to a story on TikTok about them. She read as much as she could about them. It didn't make her feel less like she was going to float into the sky, but it made her feel less alone. Less crazy. Sarah worked at Target until she saved up enough money for her apartment. And she knew the moment she walked inside that she would never want to leave again.

I told Sarah that it made perfect sense that she didn't want to leave her house.

She laughed. "That's what my therapist said—she told me, 'Sarah, the world hasn't been good to you, and it's a very scary place, so why wouldn't it be out to get you?'"

"And that includes the sky," Sarah added. "It's just everything around us, even the things that we would normally maybe think are innocuous, like nature or clouds or something. Which sucks because before this all happened to me, I loved nature. I love everything about it. Nature was my God."

Sarah paid a neighbor $150 a month to take out her trash and get her mail. Every other week, he also bought her vapes at the gas station. Once a month he grabbed her meds from Walgreens. If she had an emergency or a bad UTI, she tipped a DoorDash driver. Sometimes the ladies in the office brought her the mail, but not all the time. All her doctor's appointments were telehealth. All her groceries were delivered.

She cooked lobster cheddar casserole or crab rangoon stuffed salmon. One day she made a Twix frappuccino and dyed her hair black. She ate leftover chicken out of a Cool Whip container and watched *Jumanji* and then made $10 on phone sex. She did phone sex or video sex. Phone sex was easier because it didn't require dressing up or putting on long fake lashes. On slow days she might make $160 a night. Some nights she made $1,000. On really slow days she'd bring in $40. If men asked, What do you want? and she said, I want your money, then she knew it was time to be done for the day.

Most nights she had the same dream: about a big castle with a lot of different rooms. This castle was her home. She had a bird's-eye view of the castle, and it was huge. One time a meteor struck the castle, and it disintegrated into nothing.

When Sarah was a kid her family lived in Las Vegas for a few years while her mom worked night shifts at the casinos. Those nights, Sarah told me, her mom sometimes left her at home alone to look after her little sister. At the time, Sarah was only six years old. She often stayed in her bedroom with the doors locked because she was sure that if she left the room, someone was going to hurt her. One time she peered out the window and saw a man looking up at her with binoculars. He looked like a bug. It was her mother's stalker. He had been stalking them for a few months: lingering outside their apartment, leaving gifts by the door, trailing their car on the road.

Now in Omaha, Sarah was afraid of the dark again, just as she had been as a child. Especially in the summers, when there were a lot of crickets, which her cat killed and left the bodies on the ground. She was haunted by memories of men and violence, stalkers and intruders, and her paranoia took the form of a large cricket, looking for her, showing up at her window. She knew that if she looked out the window, the cricket would look back at her.

"I had to close my bedroom door at night because I would roll over and look out my door and swear to God I saw the cricket standing there," Sarah told me.

"How long were you afraid of the big cricket?" I asked.

"I was afraid of the big cricket for a month," she said.

"Was it a cricket that was going to kill you?" I said.

"He was going to beat me up really, really bad with all his little hands. That's what I was envisioning. It was bad. These thoughts that I have, they make no sense. They're literally not plausible. If I step outside, am I going to fly off the face of the earth? Is a cloud going to come down and crush me? Absolutely not. When I'm in that moment, you can't convince me otherwise. You can't."

Recently, Sarah pushed herself to drive to Hy-Vee to get some groceries. When she got to the parking lot, she was breathing heavily and her body was shaking so bad the brake pedal came loose. "I was having a panic attack. I was like, Fuck this. I can't go into the store like this. Everyone's going to be looking at me. I'm going to be so embarrassed. I can't do this."

She drove away and ran a red light and then pulled over in the middle of the intersection to vomit because she was so anxious about running the red light. She could barely keep her hands on the wheel the rest of the way because of all the shaking. She got out of the car and sprinted to her building. Once inside, the panic was gone. "I always tell people agoraphobia is the avoidance of fear," she told me. "The fear of fear itself. We're so afraid to feel fearful that we avoid anything that triggers the fear, to our own detriment."

She really did hope to leave one day. She was doing well up until last spring, when she made it to the other side of her building and then relapsed.

"I've come a long way," she said, "even if it doesn't seem like it to a lot of people. I can go out and get my groceries from a driver's car. I can meet my driver at the building door. Now I can get in the shower with my oven going. I can even look out the windows," she told me. "But I can't look for too long."

Home was a place to recover from all the ways her trust had been betrayed by other human beings, and she was going to build that trust back, slowly, over time.

But for now, Sarah misses going into stores and running into people she knows. She misses smelling candles and being able to pick her own produce. She misses being inconvenienced by other people. She misses seeing wildflowers and hearing children laugh. She misses eavesdropping on conversations in stores. She misses swimming. She misses going to the movie theater when it's really hot outside and feeling really cold once she gets inside. She misses seeing friends. She misses animals and plants. She misses the smell of a gas station in the rain. She misses driving around at night listening to music, walking in nature and looking out into the distance and not expecting anything and being suddenly overwhelmed by beauty.

"I feel like, with everything that I've been through, I should be able to overcome agoraphobia. I shouldn't be afraid of the sun or of the sky. I've been through much worse. I've literally been kidnapped. I've literally been raped. I've had guns pointed at me. I've been stabbed. I shouldn't be afraid of the sun. I struggle with that. And I feel like I'm a loser, to be honest. I feel like I'm a loser."

The "primary feature of agoraphobia," feminist geographer Joyce Davidson wrote, "is its impact on the boundaries of the embodied self." This includes losing one's place in space and time, confusing borders between what is outside and inside the body.

Davidson's agoraphobic women seemed to have lost a sense of being contained within the boundaries of their own bodies—suddenly vulnerable to the outside world. These women's bodies felt "unbounded," as if they were disappearing, exploding, or crumbling, fluid and unfixed on earth. The historian Susan Bordo, an agoraphobic, also recalled feeling substance-less: "a medium through which body, breath, and world would rush."

In Davidson's research, a sufferer named Ruth explained, "I feel as though there's no . . . no top of my head. I feel as though it's all opened up, and it's air . . . as if there's wind or something." For some, agoraphobic panic makes them feel as if they are being pulled into an abyss. Their own bodies are not enough to keep themselves safe. They might also have feelings of being unreal or far away, have weakness in their limbs or a sensation of faintness or falling.

To keep themselves in their body, it helped to remind themselves that they had one. A sufferer named Susan explained how she used to take her house keys and dig them into her hand. "You know, a wee bit of short sharp shock treatment." And there was another woman who snapped a rubber band on her wrist. They needed to know that their bodies were their own and not the world's to take. Pain helped them define their boundaries.

If they ventured outside, these agoraphobics looked for solid things to hide behind or hold on to: lampposts, benches, trees, a companion, a stick, or an umbrella. Wearing a hat or sunglasses was helpful for some. Others felt safer hiding behind a newspaper, pushing a stroller, or having a child around. Stormy days were better than sunny ones. Cars were often safe as they were extensions of home. The novelist Ford Madox Ford managed to cross Salisbury Plain by moving quickly from bench to bench.

Reddit user Sunflower Bitch wrote in an Ask Me Anything forum, "I often don't even leave my room unless I absolutely have to. That's the only time that I don't feel eyes on me." She lives on the outskirts of a small town in the Midwest, and it's quiet, but occasionally she hears a train or a couple of cars pass by. Sunflower Bitch thinks she was conditioned to self-isolate as a child and taught to pick a safe spot when things were bad.

"I was left alone for a long time laying in my bed and staring at the ceiling . . . I needed permission most of the time to even leave."

QUESTION: If you were to be put in something constraining like a Darth Vader suit, would you be able to venture outside of your property without issue?

SUNFLOWER BITCH: I don't think so. Half of my issue is feeling like I am being watched when stepping outside. That would just draw more attention to me.

QUESTION: What if you were to go to a Star Wars convention wearing said Darth Vader suit, where you would blend in, would that still be a problem for you?
SUNFLOWER BITCH: In that scenario, I might be able to do that.

I've never been agoraphobic, but I remember the first time I had the sense that the boundaries of my body were being invaded. It wasn't a virus or a worm or a wound packed with dirt but the fear of inheriting Nana's fanaticism. When Nana hugged me, I always felt the particular urge to brush away the area of contact, trying to define a barrier between us.

It reminded me of the women who talked about feeling a man's violation under their skin and inside the body, diffuse and hard to locate, not just on the surface. How their skin was not enough of a barrier to keep them safe.

Roxane Gay writes about keeping herself safe in the aftermath of sexual violence by making her body like "a fortress, impermeable." In *Hunger: A Memoir of (My) Body,* Gay writes: "I ate and ate and ate in the hopes that if I made myself big, my body would be safe. . . . I was trapped in my body, one that I barely recognized or understood, but at least I was safe." She had built her own walls, felt guarded by her own body—another kind of home.

When agoraphobia was first named by Carl Westphal in 1871, all his patients were men. Staying inside the home in nineteenth-century Europe was pathological for men but not women. In fact, a woman out alone in public was assumed to be a prostitute. The spread of venereal diseases at the time made prostitutes, and by default other public women, dangerous. Syphilis, which caused neurological issues, was on the rise, and it was assumed that promiscuity, not disease, drove women to insanity. Ideas about prostitutes meant women who worked late shifts risked their reputation just by walking home from work.

This is all to say that the associations between "insanity" and "outside women" were firmly planted in the public's imagination and fed the assumption that women who were harassed, assaulted, or raped should have known better than to be outside the home.

Freud had treated a few agoraphobics himself. When a five-year-old boy called Little Hans witnessed a horse falling and became too afraid to go out into the streets, Freud believed it was because he was deeply alarmed by the size of the horse's penis. Freud thought agoraphobia was about repressed anxieties in men, while for women agoraphobia depended on "a romance of prostitution," meaning agoraphobic women feared their own sexuality, and would go wild outside, having sex with random men on the streets.

After World War I, when it was permissible for women to go outside unescorted, the number of agoraphobic women rose. "Women who were originally prohibited by law and custom from entering public areas," wrote sociologist Joy B. Reeves, "are now diagnosed as phobic when participation in the public arena makes them unduly anxious."

The essayist Nancy Mairs became agoraphobic soon after she married and had children. "There's nothing like the symptoms of agoraphobia for keeping a woman in her place," she wrote. In a study of the husbands of agoraphobic women, the husbands suffered when their wives recovered. They became depressed and anxious, occasionally suicidal. They described feeling abandoned or suddenly inadequate when their wives started work or went out to socialize. One husband developed a severe psychogenic pain disorder.

In fact, several studies found that more than half of non-agoraphobic women actually scored in the clinical range for agoraphobia. In other words, just being raised female was enough to qualify for a clinical diagnosis.

———

One California winter, late in the pandemic, when days of heat plunged to cold at night, I visited family outside Los Angeles. The house was among eucalyptus trees and lizards with forked tails and an invasive plant that was bright orange and beautiful but strangled any plants in its way. In the morning, a red-tailed hawk with fluffy legs napped in the trees.

I was in pain as usual. My hip ached, and I tensed my shoulders until the muscles hardened and yanked a nerve in my spine. A friend recommended a woman named Tonnia. Because of the pandemic, she came to people's homes with a massage table strapped to her back. "People always call me Dora the Explorer," she said.

I undressed and slipped under dark green sheets. "Being human is hard," she said. "I say that all the time." She touched my shoulders, dug her fingers between muscles with long names. "It's like a beaver dam in here," she said. "You have to get back in your body. You're not in your body."

She had been the same way, she told me. Tense and anxious. It got so bad that she couldn't leave her home for two years. "I was too afraid," she said.

Tonnia wasn't sure what she was afraid of, but at night she always woke up having a panic attack. Her boyfriend would just roll over and stare at her in the dark before silently rolling back over to sleep. This was in Sacramento in 2014. At the time, she couldn't keep her eyes still—they were moving around and looking at everything. All she could think about was death. It wasn't like a car was going to hit her or she was going to get struck by lightning, nothing like that. It simply felt like she was going to die. At the emergency room, where she ended up after her attacks, they always asked, "Do you feel an impending sense of doom?" And she always said yes. They gave her Ativan and she slept for days and it made her feel like a zombie and she didn't want to be a zombie, so she stopped going to the emergency room and stopped taking Ativan.

Instead, Tonnia worked longer hours at her job to distract herself, letting her thoughts disappear into the sinews and knots of the human body. Her office was the only place she felt safe. She wanted to leave her house but didn't know how to fix herself. She couldn't afford therapy and had no insurance.

"I truly can't think of any particular traumatic events that caused it," she said. Then she remembered not just one moment but many instances that made her afraid to leave her house, and most of them involved penises.

At her first job at a spa in Roseville, a man flipped over on the table with a boner. Sometimes that happened and she didn't want to embarrass the man, so she always waited a moment, but this man didn't say anything—didn't apologize—and the boner didn't go away. She noticed it was moving. "The thing was moving around," she said. "Like, it was flying around."

She asked her boyfriend, "Why was it moving around? Why didn't it go away? When you have a boner, can you move it around?"

He didn't know what she meant.

She asked the same question, only louder. "When you have a boner, can you flex it and move it around?"

"Yeah," he said. "Totally."

She decided that client was flagging her down with his penis.

There were lots of stories like this one. Just yesterday one of Tonnia's clients told her how a male massage therapist tucked the sheet into the top of her panties and then "took off the sheet and gave her a wedgie, and then massaged her butt cheeks, both at the same time, just like spreading her hoo-ha out." The woman told Tonnia she froze and she knew that it was wrong and she should say something but she just couldn't.

While Tonnia was working at Massage Envy, a man wafted the sheet up as if he needed air on his body, and started pushing the sheet down, and down, until it was below his waist "so his cock and balls were out but no boner." She took her hands off him and stood at the back of the table and waited for him to realize his mistake and to say that he was sorry, or else to tell her "to suck it or something," and then she could tell him to leave. But he didn't say anything. She wanted to give him a chance, but when he didn't cover his cock and balls, she told him the massage was over.

Will you wear lingerie?

Will you tickle my toes?

Men texted her about all kinds of things. They texted her about the kinds of massages that she had to look up even to know what they were talking about. For example: You're naked and there's lots of oil and you're using the client's body as a

Slip'n Slide and your body as a massage tool, just boobs and body slipping and sliding.

One client texted: I just need you to tell me it's okay for me to masturbate. I just feel really guilty and I just need you to tell me it's okay for me to do this.

Goodbye, she said.

I just finished anyway, he said.

Tonnia was a new therapist experiencing these things for the first time, and now she was too scared to massage a man. "And that's when I started having these panic attacks," she explained. She removed her photo from her website, hoping to mitigate any assumption that pleasuring them was part of her job. In case things got bad, she carried certain tools with her.

"One's very long and steel and I could definitely fuck somebody up with that. And the other you hold like brass knuckles. If I punched someone in the throat with that, I could kill them."

The very first time she saw an unwanted penis she was ten years old and walking home from school. A baby-blue Falcon pulled to the curb. The driver had blond greasy hair that fell to his shoulders and a clown-white face, almost as if caked in makeup. And his penis was out. He coasted alongside her as she walked. This was in Phoenix, on Cholla Street, and he cruised around the neighborhood flashing his penis at neighborhood kids for seven or eight years. In high school, she remembered how he cut her off in the middle of the road and started to get out of the car. And she sprinted to a neighbor's house and the girl who lived there said she knew about him too. Tonnia never told her mom about it.

The first time she was able to leave her house was when one of her clients invited her to an all-women's Mary Kay makeup party. "At that moment, I remembered feeling like, This is safe. It's all women. It's safe, and that was the first time I left my house."

In recent months, Tonnia got on the dating apps and chatted with a guy. She gave him her number.

"We were flirty, and all of a sudden he sends me a video of him stroking his fucking penis and he's like, 'You want to be Daddy's little cum slut?'"

It wasn't time, she thought. Or maybe it was okay, maybe the world would always be a little bit scary. She had plans. She was going to collect all those messages and put them into a book so people would know. "It's not just the women with bruises walking around," she told me. "It's the ones that seem fine I'm thinking about."

Meditation was the only thing that she could do to relax, because it was free and because she didn't have to leave home. At first she hated it—it made her want to scream and jump out of her skin. She could go for a minute. Then two minutes. Then five. Slowly, she felt better, less plagued by anxiety. After about a year she could meditate for hours and hours.

"It's my favorite place to be," she told me. In such a state, she had visions and dreams. Once, she thought she got up to talk to the television, but when she turned around she saw herself on the sofa meditating. She had a vision of a woman with pale skin and bright red hair swooping in on her right side, putting her face in Tonnia's. "Whatever this is," Tonnia had said, "I'm not ready for that." She understood this as a new power she had gained through suffering. She thought she was getting messages.

———

My habits of self-preservation didn't keep me indoors, but they did leave me frozen and immobile.

A memory of when I'm thirteen or fourteen: I'm way out in eastern Oregon, where it's all desert, and I'm sitting in a pickup truck waiting for my mother. We are parked in the dirt lot of a general store. She's inside, buying snacks. When I roll down the window to clear away a layer of dust, I find myself face-to-face with a leathery man. Fluffy gray hair sits atop his head like smoke. He leans against a wooden post and grins. I do not move—I cannot move. I study a pattern of wrinkles on the car's faux leather seat. He stands a good fifteen feet away on the porch of the general store, but I'm trapped in his gaze until my mother arrives. I jolt awake and dip my hands into the grocery bag. I tear into a Cheetos bag.

How do I look when I am afraid? Perfectly fine. And that's one of the more difficult things.

The Frozen Ones

A TWENTY-YEAR-OLD COLLEGE WOMAN GOES WITH HER friends to a frat party and meets a guy. She likes him. They are flirting among the plastic chairs, the beer cups, the Miller Lite boxes. He says, Do you want to go back to one of the bedrooms? She does. They mess around, but they don't have sex. She doesn't want to have sex. But when he tries, she's like, No, no, no, I don't know you. He uses his elbows to pin her down and that's when she freezes, and she stays completely frozen throughout the rape.

When he finishes, he gets up and notices that she's still just lying there, and so he goes out and tells all his friends, Hey, I just had sex with so-and-so and she's still there!

The men line up on the porch to take turns going into the bedroom to sexually assault her. The woman is conscious but can't move, even after the first man leaves and a second man steps in to harm her.

She's just lying there, one man after another.

This is all happening ten feet away from where other people are hanging out. A friend overhears people bragging about raping the girl who won't move, and she barges into the bedroom. She shakes her friend, trying to get her to snap out of it. But she won't move—it's like lifting a dead body. After she's dragged off the bed, the frozen woman suddenly starts moving again.

She is taken to the hospital. The nurses do a medical exam and a forensic evidence collection kit, and file a police report. The police refuse to pick up the kit. There were just too many men involved. A "sloppy mess," they call it. And so they close the case.

Rebecca Campbell shared this story at a 2012 lecture at the National Institute of Justice. Campbell is a psychologist and professor at Michigan State University who studies institutional responses to sexual violence. She learned about the case during a ten-year research project that investigated why so many sexual-assault cases reported to the police are rarely prosecuted.

Campbell interviewed the victim and her friends, as well as the police officer who closed the case. When Campbell asked the officer why he stopped the investigation, he told her, "No one wants to have a train pulled on them, so if she just laid there and took it, she must have wanted it."

"There is another explanation," Campbell told the crowd at the National Institute of Justice. "The explanation is tonic immobility."

Or "thanatosis," the ancient Greek word for preparing for death.

A year before I learned about the work of Rebecca Campbell, I came across a peculiar video of an opossum pretending to be dead. The opossum was in a barn with two birds and a frog, also playing dead. These paralyzed bodies struck me as familiar—reminding me of some general feeling I had about being a woman in the world. I watched the video again and again.

A friend once told me she'd played dead when she was sexually assaulted. I didn't know what she meant. But after watching videos of animals playing dead, I learned they were paralyzed against their will by an ancient evolutionary response to the threat of predation known as thanatosis, or tonic immobility. Maybe she *couldn't* move? Maybe it wasn't giving up: It was shutting down.

I went looking for someone who had experienced this kind of immobility in response to sexual assault, and that's how I met Lee, who was nineteen when she was raped during a military exercise a few summers earlier. "I just froze," she told me.

It had been a long, hot day of training—marching into the hills, carrying heavy packs, eating MREs. Lee's group had been honing their navigation skills, figuring out how to get from one place to another as quickly as possible with only a compass and points, all while avoiding ambushes and snakes.

That night, she fell asleep and woke up to a man lying next to her—touching her with his finger before raping her. "I felt like I wanted to scream or yell or push him," she told me. "And I don't even know why, but my body just wouldn't react." At some point after he finished, she could move again. The man left her side, and she fell back asleep, though she doesn't remember when.

The next morning she ate breakfast and immediately threw it up. She couldn't understand her failure to respond to the attack. It felt at odds with her training—the hours she had spent learning how to survive and fight against all kinds of threats. When she was a child, her mother would say, You're a girl, and you're small, so you're an easy target. She listened to her mother's warning and took pride in herself for being competitive and athletic. She played basketball, baseball, football, and soccer, and she ran cross-country. She was sometimes on men's teams. "No one expects to be a victim of such a situation," she said. "But everyone imagines how they would react, and I had always imagined I would fight and get away."

She was ashamed of herself for not doing anything. "Because it's not really who I am," she said.

While scanning the news, I noticed a Lingua Franca that women were using, a repeated vocabulary to describe what they experienced and thought during a sexual assault, and variations of the word "freezing" are most often part of that vocabulary. I started collecting examples of this language.

In 2019, a forty-eight-year-old woman testified in a Canadian court that she "froze" when a man raped her in the back of his car after their first date. A victim of a sexual-assault case in Australia said in court that she would never forget being "practically naked and frozen on a massage table."

The Norwegian actress and model Natassia Malthe reported being "a dead person" when she was raped. In an episode of the documentary series *The Me You Can't See,* Lady Gaga describes being raped at nineteen: "I just froze." And so did actress Gabrielle Union when she was raped at a gas station as a teen.

"I just absolutely froze," Brooke Shields said in the documentary *Pretty Baby*, describing how she felt when being raped. "I just thought, Stay alive and get out."

"I'm not a screamer," E. Jean Carroll testified at the U.S. District Court in Manhattan about how Donald Trump sexually abused her in a dressing room at Bergdorf Goodman. She told the court she was "too much in a panic to scream." Miriam Haley, a former production assistant on *Project Runway*, testified that when Harvey Weinstein held her down and forced himself on her, "I was in so much shock at the time that I just checked out."

In an article for *Vice*, the writer Jackie Hong wrote of her rape, "When he started pulling down my pants and underwear, my body seemed to freeze over."

"As soon as he grabbed my ass," Taylor Swift stated in a July 2016 court deposition against former radio DJ David Mueller, "I became shocked and withdrawn and was barely able to say 'Thanks for coming,' which is what I say to everybody. I was barely able to get the words out, and it was like somebody switched the lights off in my personality."

Most of the news was focused on the assaults of celebrities, so I started interviewing ordinary people who were also survivors of sexual assault and paying close attention to patterns in their language. I spoke to dozens of women, and they also talked about their experiences in terms of freezing. Andrea Royer, a yoga instructor, told me that when she was attacked in September 2012 in Spearfish, South Dakota, she fought and screamed to deter her rapist, but eventually she "froze" because she decided "freezing" was the only way she could keep herself alive.

A seventy-five-year-old women's rights activist named Joyce Short used "freezing" to describe her response to being strangled by the man who ultimately raped her as a college student. "The more I struggled," she said, "the more he pressed on my neck." She was having trouble breathing, so she stopped struggling and pretended to be unconscious to survive.

When Jenna Sorenson said she "froze," she meant she acquiesced to the sex because he was on top of her, and it was going to happen no matter what. He was a bodybuilder—and she had just dumped him. She was sure he was going to kill her, and he almost did. After he strangled her, she took a photo of the way the blood leaked into the whites of her eyes.

Samantha Woods, a Navy veteran in Florida, didn't say no, not with her body or her voice, because she was thinking about how she didn't have a ride home and how he would leave her in the parking lot and how he might have a weapon and it was better to be safe than to be in a car with a man and his gun.

The women seemed to talk about freezing both as a strategy they used to stay alive, as well as a response that was outside their control.

A few weeks later I read a victim statement by Jessica Mann, an actress who testified that Harvey Weinstein had raped her. In the statement, Mann wanted to clarify her own account of freezing—because, she said, "so many women, myself included, have only been able to find words such as 'I gave up' or 'I lost control' and, like myself, 'I froze.'"

Mann cited a 2015 paper in the *Harvard Review of Psychiatry* on the automatic defense behaviors of humans and animals, explaining that when Weinstein raped her, she experienced symptoms consistent with an extreme response to threat known as tonic immobility, which renders victims unable to scream or move their limbs.

"I ask you to consider the horrors of being rendered immobile by my own biological response," she told the court, "while I had to endure his penis, raping me on his time, as slow as he wanted while he pleasured himself inside my body. I wish I had been able to fight him while he raped me."

Mann stressed the confusion this reaction caused her—for not having a "bodily response that fought back." Since she believed she should have resisted, her shame made her prone to depression and post-traumatic stress.

. . .

What is tonic immobility? It's a temporary catatonic state that draws its evolutionary power from the fact that many predators seem hardwired to lose interest in dead prey, as their meat could harbor deadly bacteria.

The response is often triggered by restraint, or when escape seems impossible, like the moment a squirrel is gripped by the talons of a hawk. Muscles go stiff, resembling rigor mortis. The body is numbed and extremities might tremble. It's an act of self-preservation that evolved to give prey one last chance at survival and to alleviate the agony and horror of being eaten alive. Animals may whimper, whereas humans can't speak, even if they try.

For more than a century, scientists studied this phenomenon in animals, and over the years it's been named and renamed— animal hypnosis, animal magnetism, death feigning, playing dead, apparent death, and thanatosis.

Women, it seemed, were responding to rape in the same manner as immobilized prey animals.

Opossums are peaceful and slow-moving prey—and they are also nature's best death feigners. To mimic death the opossum leaves its mouth open in a toothy grin, tongue flopped to the ground, a small paw turned to the sky. Its heart rate drops by nearly half, respiration by a third. It farts a foul-smelling mucus.

The hognose snake is more theatrical—he spurts blood from his nostrils and dances before going into corpse-mode. The leaf-litter frog goes belly up, shuts its eyes, and stretches its legs in an imitation of rigor mortis.

Some female dragonflies play dead to avoid mating. They plummet from the sky and remain motionless on the ground until the males are gone. While most animals experience immobility as an act of self-preservation, California orcas are thought to weaponize the response by flipping over young great white sharks, inducing immobility for so long the sharks suffocate.

What's wrong with me? This was the first question Moriah Schiewe asked after she was raped during her first year of law school at DePaul University. Her memories of the assault were vivid, but she did not remember physical pain despite all the bruises on her thighs. But more frightening was the paralysis. She could not move any of her muscles and she could not speak or scream. But why would that be? That wasn't something that happened to people, as far as she knew.

One night, unable to sleep, her laptop screen glowing in the dark, she started googling things like "paralysis," "assault," and "numb." She found stories about animals playing dead. She found videos of hypnotized chickens, death-feigning snakes, rigid opossums, and sharks going belly up in a trance. These animals reminded Schiewe of what had happened to her. But could it be? She started to go deeper into her research until she saw full-body paralysis was a common response to sexual assault. It was depressing.

Why were women googling animal videos to understand their responses to rape?

Tonic immobility is most commonly reported in sexual-assault cases, though it's rarely discussed, and the same response has been reported in testimonies from soldiers on the front lines of war and victims of torture, natural disasters, exploding oil platforms, car crashes, and animal attacks. I found an American soldier's account of tonic immobility in the *Harvard Review of Psychiatry*, describing how during his first firefight in Iraq, "he was unable to lift his head, move his limbs, or aim his rifle." He recalled "a heavy sensation that he could not resist." He couldn't respond to his commander's orders. A comrade repeatedly hit the immobilized soldier's helmet until he was able to move again.

Sunda TeBockhorst is a practicing psychologist in Colorado who began researching tonic immobility among sexual-assault victims more than twenty years ago. She found that victims who lacked a language or framework to understand their immobility often make their own meanings with narratives of blame. For some, she observed, as soon as the assault began, they started wondering what others would say and think about them. And some women who had experienced tonic immobility during a sexual assault continued to experience tonic immobility in the future, even when they tried to have consensual sex with their partners. In almost all of these cases, their partners were not aware that it was happening, and the women didn't tell them either because they didn't have the language, or they were too ashamed. "They had to try to grin and bear it and muscle through it," TeBockhorst told me.

Veronique Valliere is a forensic psychologist often called to help explain to judges and jurors why victims don't resist or try to escape—including in high-profile cases like Bill Cosby's. When the defense tries to say that the victim didn't fight back "so she must have wanted it," Valliere will explain that no one "lying there paralyzed" is a consensual sexual partner. "If you're having sex with someone who's frozen in place," she told me, "then you're assaulting them, because that person is not into it. Any human being would know that."

She's also talked to offenders who say, Well, I thought she wanted it because she was just lying there.

"We need to understand that freezing is involuntary from a

medical and scientific perspective in order to change the perception that it is a failure of agency," she told me. "In terms of volition, tonic immobility is no different than having a severed spinal cord."

———

The weeks that followed Lee's rape were exhausting, especially with the demands of military training on top of the stress of the assault. There were sleepless nights and meals she couldn't stand to eat. She lost twenty pounds. Friends had to feed her bites of bread to make sure she was consuming enough calories.

She always used to sleep on her side, but she no longer felt safe in that position. If she did fall asleep, it was for only an hour or two before she woke up again in tears. Her heart raced, and her sheets were soaked with sweat. "I felt like I couldn't trust my own body," she said.

When friends and mentors found out how she responded during the rape, they were appalled and confused. You didn't do anything? You didn't say anything? You froze? "It didn't even feel like I could do anything," she recalled. "I wanted to scream. I was trying to scream, but it felt like I couldn't." It was difficult to explain, she said. It made her question whether she had the capability to be a leader. What if she froze again?

She knew she needed help, but she was afraid to talk to a psychologist because of the stigma around mental health programming in the military. When she couldn't sleep, she stepped outside her shared dorm room to read in the hallway in an effort to make sense of her situation. She perused articles and self-help books such as *The Body Keeps the Score* and *The Rape Recovery Handbook*, and she was upset to learn it might take her whole life to recover. She was in so much physical, mental, and emotional anguish she did not think that time was a solution at all. The nausea, the inability to remember or process information, the disconnect from her peers and friends: "I felt incredibly different. Like I never belonged with my peers again. And everyone wants to feel like they belong." It all added up. Years later, the pain became less intense, as friends said it would, but a certain joy she'd once had about life seemed permanently gone.

Months after the assault, she finally spoke with a counselor, who explained to her that "freezing" was a normal response to assault, but she didn't get much more information other than a comparison to being "like a deer caught in the glare of headlights." Her peers talked a lot about fight or flight as it related to the enemy on the field, but she didn't remember them ever talking about freezing. She heard about soldiers who froze up during battle, and she knew the shame attached to it because it made them appear weak or cowardly.

Several months after the attack, she had a nightmare. "I was waking up to the assault happening just as it had happened, and my lips were glued or sewn shut." The imagery of the dream perfectly illustrated her experience: "In my head, I was screaming. But my body wouldn't move."

It's statistically uncommon for somebody to physically fight back during a sexual assault. Verbal resistance is more common, but even that occurs less often than people imagine. "And yet victims," Jim Hopper told me, "beat up on themselves for not fighting or fleeing."

Hopper is a clinical psychologist and teaching associate at Harvard Medical School who has been studying the neurobiology of fear in sexual-assault victims for more than thirty years. Hopper studies what happens to the brain of a victim during an assault, rather than in the aftermath. "Survivors should be able to use whatever language they want," said Hopper. "But if we're going to be professionals, we need to have more precise language that's based on what's actually going on in the brain and how these things can play out."

In everyday speech, "freezing"—as scientists use the term— is often conflated with tonic immobility, but they are not the same.

Whether human or animal, the brain's first response to threat is always to stop moving. Within a fraction of a second, physiological changes prime the body for fighting or fleeing, but in sexual-assault victims, Hopper explained, this most commonly leads to involuntary freezing, where victims are motionless but attentive to threat. Or they might be able to move around and talk, but it will be difficult to think or make rational decisions. Freezing tends to come early in an attack, and extreme responses like tonic immobility typically come later, but they can happen in any order. Shifts between behaviors occur in milliseconds.

"One of the cruelest things about tonic immobility," he told me, "is if you're not dissociating, you can be all too aware of what's happening in your body, but you're utterly helpless to do anything about it."

And there's more: Hopper once worked on a case in which a man tried to force a victim to perform oral sex, but she couldn't hold her head up. "She reported that her neck muscles were totally limp, and her head literally flopped around," he said. It's called collapsed immobility, another extreme response, involving a precipitous drop in heart rate and blood pressure, causing limp muscles—unlike the rigid muscles of tonic immobility. Victims might describe the experience with phrases like "I felt dizzy," "I felt faint," or "I felt sleepy." Some victims describe this as "blacking out," which can result in untrained investigators thinking the victim drank too much alcohol.

Some people threatened with rape will acquiesce because they believe it will help them avoid severe physical injury or death, which can also look like freezing. Others fight or flee, and some won't experience a trauma response at all. But all these responses can have profoundly different effects on people's consciousness and memory, which shapes the way they tell stories about what happened to them.

Neuroscientists often talk about the brain in terms of circuitries, collections of connected areas responsible for certain functions. The defense circuitry is one of the best studied, and it works in the same basic way in all mammals: If a threat is detected, the defense circuitry can dominate brain functioning, with major consequences for logic, behavior, and memory. It takes up to three seconds for the defense circuitry to seriously impair the prefrontal cortex, and once this part of the brain goes quiet, so does our ability to reason. Our language centers are impaired. Our attention changes, and so does the way we encode memories.

Amy Arnsten, a neuroscientist at Yale University, is one of the leading researchers on the way stress impairs the prefrontal cortex. Her team recently found that exposure to even mild but uncontrollable stress quickly impaired the prefrontal cortex in humans and animals. "Under stress, your brain disconnects from its more recently evolved circuits and strengthens many of the primitive circuits, and then these unconscious reflexes that are very ancient kick in," she told me over the phone.

Arnsten described walking through the woods in Vermont some years ago when a bear dropped out of a tree. Without thinking, she froze. The bear looked at her but didn't see her.

"It just is a reflex," she said. "Most animals see movement and not detail, so freezing—especially if you're in a position where you can't escape—has had survival value across the eons."

Arnsten added that when we are under chronic stress, we actually lose gray matter in the prefrontal cortex over time. We lose it in the very corridor that's used for recently evolved circuits to control more primitive circuits. "And one of the things that's been shown is that people who've had lesions in this corridor, due to strokes or a tumor, are much more vulnerable to misinformation." So chronic stress or traumatic experiences can make us more likely to misread signs of danger—or even join a cult.

After reading testimonies of rape victims over the course of a decade, Jim Hopper observed that sometimes victims will experience what he calls "shocked freezing," when a person's mind can stay blank for several seconds; and victims might describe this with phrases like "I couldn't even think" or "I had no idea what to do." A state of impaired deliberation that Hopper calls "no-good-choices freezing" may follow, when victims find their ability to think seriously diminished. They may have trouble remembering practical information, like the fact that there are people nearby who could hear them scream.

Even if brain functions are impaired, victims can still "look" normal: They might be talking or moving around. But then they'll make compromised decisions. Hopper understands this as a kind of "freezing" too. Hopper sees it all the time in sexual assaults that happen during a massage session. "They don't think to turn over or say no or to get up and leave. They think they have to run down the hallway naked and screaming, which no one wants to do, and so usually they don't do anything because they can't think of a better option."

Then Hopper said something that shocked me. At some point during a sexual assault, or while being harassed, most victims revert to habits, usually passive or submissive ones, that have been conditioned by culture or abuse, sexism or racism. The brain is hijacked just enough for us to fall back on whatever we've been conditioned to do. "Even movements involved in sex acts might be automatically generated habits designed to please," Hopper told me. For women, this too often means being nice, trying not to bruise a man's ego, or trying to de-escalate. "And these are actually among the most common automatic responses that people have while being sexually assaulted," Hopper said. "We usually don't think of these habits as involuntary, but they absolutely are."

Hopper's insight reminded me of some papers I'd read about the impact of gender conditioning on fear behavior. The science tells us that taking on stereotypical female gender roles can increase feelings of fear and anxiety, can make us evaluate traumatic events as more threatening and uncontrollable, can make us have more intense emotional responses, can increase the likelihood that we will dissociate, or cope with avoidance, or imagine alternative outcomes. And all of these factors can heighten the impact of traumatic events.

Hopper, for example, once testified at a trial of a senior officer accused of the rape of a young Marine. The woman said the officer attacked her after a party, holding her down and ripping off her clothes. The defense argued that the Marine's military training would make it impossible for her to be raped. Hopper testified that even well-conditioned habits don't necessarily carry over from one context to another. It's why the military spends a lot of money training soldiers in realistic environments. Hopper explained that the Marine was not fighting an enemy on a battlefield, so her military training didn't kick in. Instead, she responded the way she always did when she wanted to end unwanted advances from men: She politely asked him to stop.

———

When Lee, the military recruit, reported having been raped, the authorities she talked to didn't understand why she wouldn't have cried out when there were people nearby. In other words, they didn't believe a woman would stay quiet if a man was actually raping her.

About a year later, she had a dream that she took out a gun and shot herself. She told me, "I'm not a suicidal person, but that is probably the best way to describe how badly I felt."

In many states, prosecutors must still show that sexual contact was forced or was met with verbal or physical resistance to prove that the victim didn't consent.

"If we think of resistance as a 'no' statement or fighting back," Erin Murphy, a professor at New York University School of Law, told me, "tonic immobility is not going to work to give you a nonconsensual encounter, because in those situations the physical shutdown is not usually interpreted legally to be a 'no.'" Sometimes freezing looks like compliance. Murphy told me about cases where the woman will say she took off her skirt, for example, because it was expensive, and she didn't want to get it ripped during the assault. Among high-school- and college-age women who are sexually assaulted on dates, there's a pattern of women raising their hips just slightly to allow a man to remove their shorts. "I hear it all the time," Murphy told me about the hip lifting. "And that tiny gesture is construed as consent."

Murphy thinks there are still jurors who believe that women are responsible for freezing, and who can't recognize rape unless there was physical resistance.

In a 2009 British study of mock juries, Louise Ellison and Vanessa E. Munro looked at which rape myths could be influenced by expert testimony about victim behavior. Jurors who heard explanations for certain behaviors—a victim's lack of distress while recounting the assault at trial, say, or a delay in reporting the attack—were more likely to question why those responses were relevant to a case. But the myth that seemed most entrenched was that women would try to physically resist rape. When this myth took hold, Ellison and Munro noted, jurors were "unreceptive" to the guidance provided by experts.

In a flood of light, at the Galleria Borghese in Rome, I saw a statue of Daphne twist and leap from Apollo's grasp.

Ovid must have known something of thanatosis. To escape Apollo's lust, Daphne abandoned her human form and became a laurel tree. He wrote that a heavy numbness seized her limbs, a thick bark closed over her breast, her hair turned into leaves, her arms into branches, and her feet—so swift a moment ago— were now stuck and growing roots.

Daphne's terror looked *alive*. She was still mostly human; her transformation had just begun. Her raised hands had fully transformed into branches blooming with leaves but remained attached to the smooth flesh of human arms.

In *Metamorphoses*, women often escaped rape by transformation. Their bodies became horses, trees, lakes, reeds, frankincense. Thetis became a tigress, Philomela a nightingale, Procne a swallow. Syrinx became a reed, while Callisto turned into a bear. Cyane dissolved into a watery fountain that could no longer be held.

Dryope's metamorphosis occurred many years after she was raped by Apollo. In Ovid's tale, the transformation didn't happen until she plucked a flower, which was the nymph Lotis, who had become a plant to escape the rape of Priapus. Lotis bled human blood, even in her flower form. The blood touched Dryope, triggering a transformation into a black poplar as if to complete her escape from Apollo, mimicking the way trauma can make itself known many years after it is experienced. Roots tethered her feet to the earth and bark hardened her groin. She tore out her hair only to discover that her hands were filled with leaves. She was still a human speaking through the body of a tree until her mouth, Ovid wrote, "could say no more, could be no more."

No one in America bothered to study the psychological responses of rape victims until the early 1970s. Researchers Ann Burgess and Lynda Lytle Holmstrom observed freezing-like behaviors, what was soon termed "rape-induced paralysis," in women at Boston City Hospital. Over the course of a year, they documented that thirty-four of ninety-two patients diagnosed with "rape trauma" experienced different kinds of freezing—physically or psychologically—during their attacks. "I felt faint, trembling, and cold. . . . I went limp," one woman reported. Another said, "When I realized what he was going to do, I blanked out . . . tried not to be aware of what was going on."

Earlier studies of violated women focused exclusively on venereal diseases, pregnancy, and bodily injury. "Unlike most other 'bad events,'" writes rape historian Joanna Bourke, "which were incorporated within trauma narratives from the

1860s, the ascription of psychological trauma was only applied to rape victims a century later."

Bourke observed that in the nineteenth century women were simply expected to fend off any unwanted sexual encounters. It was assumed that a woman who didn't want to be raped would be able to muster enough force to stop it.

There is hardly any historical record of how women have named and understood their own experiences of sexual trauma. When Bourke located some of the earliest descriptions of women's psychological responses to sexual assault, "insensible" was the most common description, as well as "frigid" (a term historically used to shame sexually uptight women). According to Bourke, "insensibility" was one of the only ways women were able to justify not fighting off their attackers: A woman rendered *insensible* may not have been actually unconscious, but she was somehow out of control of her mind and body. And "insensibility" was an exemption that was only afforded to women of the upper class, or as one jurist put it, "women of undoubted character."

The psychologists Susan Suarez and Gordon Gallup argued in a 1979 article in *The Psychological Record* that immobility evolved in humans, as in other animals, as a defense against predators. They then noted how often rape convictions fell apart because victims didn't resist. "It seems ironic," they wrote, "that victims should be legally penalized for exhibiting a reaction that has such adaptive value and may be firmly embedded in the biology of our species."

In all my conversations it became increasingly apparent that freezing and tonic immobility evolved to keep humans safe from animal predators, not human ones. Unlike other animals, humans don't always lose interest if their prey looks dead; it might even make a victim more appealing.

"Sun, Moon, and Talia" by Giambattista Basile was written about sixty years before it was retold by Charles Perrault as "Sleeping Beauty." The king found Talia, the sleeper, and called out to her, but she didn't respond. She just lay there, and he "beheld her charms and felt his blood course hotly through his veins. He lifted her in his arms, and carried her to a bed, where he gathered the first fruits of love." In other words, he was turned on by a woman's unresponsive body.

Whether in a state of fight, flight, or freeze—how we look when we are afraid has historically been rendered beautiful or erotic.

"Dread made her lovely," Ovid wrote of the moment Helios raped Leucothoe.

"She was lovely even in flight," Ovid wrote of Daphne's escape from Apollo.

The French actress Emma de Caunes told *The New Yorker* about Harvey Weinstein stepping out of the shower with an erection: "The fear turns him on."

I remember looking at the painter John Millais's depiction of Ophelia, admiring her beauty, before I understood that I was looking at a woman drowning. Had I also been conditioned to see beauty this way? The model for Ophelia was Lizzie Siddal, who had bright orange hair that fell to her waist. She often posed as a dead woman for male painters of the mid-nineteenth century. In the story of Siddal's death, her husband, the poet Dante Rossetti, buried her with the only copy of some poetry he'd written. When, seven years later, he wanted the poems back, he asked his friend to dig up the grave, and Siddal was perfectly preserved, the coffin full of her long orange hair, looking just as beautiful as when she had died.

In the late 1880s in Paris, the body of a woman was supposedly pulled from the Seine at a time when it was common for the bodies of sex workers to end up in the river. Mortuary workers displayed her body in their store window, hoping that someone would identify her. No one ever did. But the workers thought she was so beautiful that before they disposed of the body they made a plaster mask of her face. The story of the corpse might be a fiction, but the idea that the mask came from a dead woman's face became part of its popular appeal. It's been mass-produced and sold as a decoration. Picasso had one. So did Rilke and Nabokov. Camus called her a "drowned Mona Lisa." She became a posthumous muse for filmmaker François Truffaut. People say she looks like she's just asleep, waiting for Prince Charming. Al Alvarez writes in *The Savage God,* "I am told a whole generation of German girls modelled their looks on her." The face of a CPR dummy is modeled after this same woman. Millions have sat at her side and kissed her rubbery lips, pretending to resuscitate her, like Sleeping Beauty. But of course, she always stays dead, which seems to be her most useful form.

When I was nineteen, I went on a trip to the Canary Islands with my friend Abby. We were living in Spain and the islands were only an hour flight from Madrid, a cheap deal we discovered on a travel website.

The afternoon we landed, we were invited to a bar by two soccer coaches whose team we'd seen practicing in a field near our hotel. The bar was empty. It didn't look like a place you were supposed to see in the daylight.

Abby drank fast, but we were drinking a lot in those days.

I sipped slow. Our Spanish wasn't perfect, but it was enough to converse. I hadn't had more than half a glass when I started to feel numb and heavy. I had trouble talking.

I remember the white of his scalp. I remember the smell of detergent, but not enough to hide the sweat. I remember the curtain more than anything, the wavy folds, the velvet fabric, the cigarette burns. That's where they made the drinks, behind that curtain browning with water stains. I could sort of move; I could barely see.

The man across from me pulled Abby close, slid his tongue into her mouth. He hoisted her out of the booth and carried her away. I tried to call out to her but couldn't. Then I felt the other man's lips. I was able to move somewhat, not entirely gone. I did push him away, and I don't remember how or when I got to the bathroom, but I found Abby on the bathroom floor, the man on top of her. I don't remember how we got back outside.

"Do you think we were drugged?" Abby asked. She didn't know why her legs didn't work. They didn't work!

At the time, we laughed about it and went back to the hotel and slept.

Immobility once belonged to the world of spells and sorcery, as a way to assert power over animals. The Egyptian snake charmers could make a cobra look dead by applying a slight pressure to the animal's neck, leaving it passive to the snake charmer's touch.

In 1646, the German scholar Athanasius Kircher believed he had induced a terrified hen into a state of enchantment by tying her feet together and holding her body and head flat on the ground. After a violent struggle, she went quiet. Kircher wrote that it was as if "she gave herself up to the will of her conqueror."

In 1778, a young German by the name of Franz Mesmer moved to Paris, dreaming of success after finding what he claimed to be a cure for a variety of common illnesses: an invisible fluid that flowed from one living body to another. The fluid, he thought, needed to be flowing for vitality. Mesmer believed he had the capacity to heal by manipulating the fluid— a process he called "animal magnetism." Most of Mesmer's patients were high-society women suffering from nervous fits or fainting spells. Mesmer had his patients sit across from him with their knees locked between his own. By staring deep into their eyes, he projected his own magnetism onto them. He touched them to find "magnetic poles." For six years Mesmer gained a cultish following in eighteenth-century France, hosting large healing sessions at his clinic. He wore a lilac silk robe and carried a magnetized iron wand, passing it over the bodies of patients who often lapsed into deep trancelike sleeps, while others convulsed in epileptic-like fits. This called for speedy transport to the so-called crisis room, where rumors of "sexual magnetism" began. The historian Robert Darnton noticed that mesmerizing was widely believed to be "a sort of sexual magic . . . and a threat to morality." Vulnerability to hypnosis was thought a form of weakness, and magnetism was a masculine force with the power to defeat a woman's will. In *Confessions of a Magnetiser*, anonymously published in 1845, the author reveals his desire to use mesmerism to control the emotions of women. Mesmer was eventually accused of sexually assaulting a nineteen-year-old girl.

––––––

The classicist Jessica Wise found one of the earliest representations of tonic immobility in Ovid's *Amores*. The narrator—the Amator—talks about sexually assaulting the courtesan Corinna and the slave Cypassis, who, because of their low social standing in Roman society, were thought immune to the fear, shame, and trauma of sexual assault. The Amator rapes the women, thinking nothing of their silence and immobility.

But what Wise discovers is Ovid's attention to the physical and emotional responses of these women. Wise notices the striking accuracy of Ovid's depictions of these responses. The women are not simply silent and passively immobile, but expressing the trauma of the experience through their bodies: paralyzed by fear and pain, unable to speak or call out. Their bodies tremble, blush, sob, and sigh. Ovid compares Corinna's apparently "lifeless limbs" to reeds shaken by the wind, ripples across the tops of waves, and a gentle breeze in the poplar. He writes of the frozen body as if it were a wilderness, deceptively quiet, but to the observant eye it's teeming with life.

Has Ovid done these women a favor by calling our attention to their expressions of fear? Wise thinks so. The women's bodies become messengers, a language for the less powerful, a mode of communicating hurt and suffering. The women's bodies expose their terror, despite everything the Amator says: that he loves them, even as he rapes them.

Rapture

MISSY ROBINSON IS A PROFESSIONAL CUDDLE THERAPIST from Australia who was sexually assaulted while training with the Australian Defence Force Academy when she was nineteen. The year was 1998, and the Academy was isolated out in the bush, with only military people living, studying, eating, and training together. She was the only woman in her section, Delta Squadron 15.

In February that year, during a training exercise, a commander started talking to her about all the things he liked when having sex. He put his hand on her thigh and stroked her leg and asked if she "liked fucking."

"I froze," she wrote of this moment in her self-published memoir. "Then the strangest thing happened. My vagina went numb. Like completely numb. So fucking weird."

Missy understood this as a warning sign—her body signaling danger. Even though her vagina seemed to have "escaped" by going numb, Missy did not. After she was raped, she ran into the bush to hide. The next week she spent in the hospital recovering from injuries.

In the days and weeks that followed, Missy didn't crumble or fall apart. "I just kept going," she told me. "Because I wanted to be an officer in the army. It was a very elite group, and I was trying to stay strong." There was a short hearing, and the commander pleaded guilty. Otherwise she didn't talk about it and didn't want anyone to know.

Missy didn't tell anyone at home about the rape either. She "tucked the memory away" to forget about it. But, about a year later, she occasionally and unconsciously acted out scenes of the violence: The first time was when she tried to fling herself out of a moving car. She was screaming and clawing at the door so the driver pulled over. Missy dashed into a swamp, and her boyfriend found her later cowering among the vegetation. Sometimes she got out a knife, "because there was a knife during the assault," and dragged the blade endlessly around the kitchen. But there was no link; everyone just dismissed it as stress.

In 2008, ten years after the rape, she was diagnosed with complex PTSD, but no one knew why because her life had been pretty nice. The link to the sexual assault didn't happen until 2018, twenty years after the fact, when she did a voluntary two-and-a-half-week stay at a private mental health facility. She was just hanging out in her room in her underwear when all of a sudden the door opened, and it was another patient: a man. "And I turned into a fucking animal," Missy told me. "I screamed at him, saying, 'Get the fuck out,' and he was like, 'Oh, I thought this was my room.'"

It was such an intense, visceral reaction that when the staff asked her what happened, she finally spoke of the incident in the bush.

The next part of her story is hard to tell because it involves hallucinations, delusions, and false memories. But one day, when she was fifteen, she found out she was pregnant, and she didn't want children. She called her mother, who offered her support and some financial assistance. She booked an appointment with a clinic and had an abortion. For six years she had this memory, and then she learned that it never happened. She was never pregnant and never went to the clinic for a procedure. But she still has the memory. "It's very hard to explain," she told me. "I wasn't lying. I wasn't making it up. In my mind, it was all happening. The psychosis had created this delusion, and I was living it."

———

I met ten-year-old Midya in a refugee camp in northern Iraq after the fall of Mosul in 2017. She had been kidnapped by the Islamic State and was now free again. She saw many dead bodies when she tried to flee into the mountains, and she was raped many times by dozens of men. It was a horrible reality and true of many children.

Even after she was safe in a refugee camp, Midya was trapped in the past, going through the motions of escape. She fainted twenty times a day, and when she did, she imagined herself falling to the ground and waking up in a beautiful forest where she was sure no one would hurt her. There were bright-feathered birds and animals who kept her safe. She spoke of extraordinary things that didn't exist in our world. Just to survive she had to leave our real world; she had to faint and fall down and dissociate. Voices spoke to her from the forest even when she was awake and moving around during the day. She talked back to them. The Iraqis called her "the girl who was always talking from another world."

"But it's normal to leave reality to survive," one of the psychiatrists at the camp, Jan Kizilhan, told me. "Unless they do, the body thinks they'll be dead. But it's a pathological way to survive. If you have to leave reality, the body will survive, but the soul will not."

The fainting was everywhere at the camp. Women falling to the ground, seeking safety, long after the fact, especially among the women who had been raped. "To avoid the rape in their minds," Kizilhan told me, "they might faint and fall down. They live with a feeling of unreality and detachment from the world."

I heard many stories like Midya's while reporting this book. The stories of women who escaped to imaginary worlds, usually in nature. There was the woman who escaped to a river and talked about the beauty of the river and the sound of the water, and didn't talk about the rape. So her story of rape was actually the story of a river. And another talked about an ancient forest, the way Midya had, and this, I thought, is how a woman becomes a tree.

———

Stacie is a petite woman in her early forties who remembers nothing of her youth. There is a gap of fourteen years, from ages five to nineteen. In those years, she was abused by her father and her stepfather, and dissociation was her escape. For a long time she thought forgetting her entire youth wasn't a big deal because when you're a kid you just don't remember much. But then she talked to other adults and realized they all had memories of their own childhoods.

Sometimes Stacie listened to stories about her life as a child, but she didn't have her own stories. Instead, Stacie collected these memories from her mother and from other people and formed a quilted narrative that resembled her youth, but was just an approximation of it. "It was weird," Stacie told me, "to hear stories about myself and have no connection to the girl in them." But over time they did come to feel like her own memories.

She did have a few memories of her own: a difficult moment from a few months she spent at a Christian boarding school for troubled youth, when a friend was unfairly targeted by one of the counselors. Stacie intervened to protect her friend. She lost her temper and felt herself rise to the ceiling, where she was stuck like a helium balloon, staring down at herself. She could see her body down below, still yelling at the counselor. When Stacie fled the room, she felt as if she were sucked back into her body. When counselors found her hiding in the forest, Stacie threw water at them. They gave her more rules to follow, and she decided, I'm out of here, bye.

Stacie's three or four other memories are about her doing chores for her stepfather or hiding from her stepfather. Her favorite hiding spot was the roof. She liked the bathroom too. Or a spot down by the river.

They didn't make a lot of videos in her family, but they had this one video of Stacie at her fifth birthday party. In the video, Stacie is a perky and engaged kid, and then suddenly, this girl in the video just stops engaging. She is somewhere else entirely. She is gone. It lasts a minute. Then her head shakes and her eyes blink and she has returned from wherever she had gone. Some sanctuary in her mind.

For a long time Stacie's mother thought her daughter was a pathological liar. She had no idea Stacie was so disconnected from reality that she might not remember her own actions. If Stacie pulled the bedroom curtains to the floor, for example, she wouldn't remember doing it. But her mother would tell her she did, and Stacie would get in trouble for it. It was anguish not having any memories, not being given the chance to understand the cause and effect of her own actions. She was constantly told that her reality wasn't real, or that she was being dramatic or misbehaving. But she was just in a different reality. If dissociation exists on a spectrum, Stacie lived with the most extreme form: dissociative identity disorder, including dissociative amnesia.

When she was nineteen, she remembered wrestling and roughhousing with her boyfriend. They were being silly. At some point she started freaking out, begging him to leave, because she didn't see her boyfriend; she only saw her stepdad. When he turned around and walked toward Stacie—playfully making as if to tackle her—she punched him in the face. Her body was going through actions in the present, but her mind was reacting to threats from the past.

Even now, when Stacie looks in the mirror, she doesn't connect to the person in the reflection. It's not that she doesn't know her face (it's not like seeing another person), but she doesn't understand her face. "How is that thing in the mirror my face? These don't feel like my hands, I'm disconnected from my hands." She touches and feels things but sometimes doesn't recognize that it is herself touching and feeling.

When she senses danger, Stacie will still immediately disconnect from the moment. "It feels like somebody turns off the light switch in a room, and I'm the light," she told me. "I disappear whether or not I want to." About five years ago, after doing work with a therapist, she started thinking about that night with her boyfriend, and wrote him a letter to thank him for not holding that punch against her over the years. But as she was writing the letter she worried the memory wasn't real. Months later, he sent her a DM on Facebook. He was happy she wrote and even apologized for egging her on.

"This was astounding," Stacie told me. "It was proof that an experience I had was real." Stacie has spent much of her life in pursuit of the real. It's why she prefers to communicate with texts, or handwritten letters, or emails, because then she has a paper trail. But really what she has been searching for is a story that makes sense for listeners who live outside the world of trauma, because of how it can change our relationships with experience and memory, giving life the feeling of unreality. And women are often wondering if the experiences they've had, of deep hurt or victimization, are "real." Maybe part of that has to do with not being believed, but I think another part has to do with the way trauma affects storytelling.

———

Traumatic events can transform our real lives into surreal experiences. Fright can render an encounter strange as it's happening as well as long after the fact. We can experience altered states, distorted perceptions, magical ideation.

I'm thinking of when I returned home to Brooklyn, after I went to Syria for a reporting trip, and I was walking around when I saw a stain of blood spread across the sidewalk. My eyes scanned for a body. When I looked back, the blood resolved into children's paint.

I was diagnosed with post-traumatic stress disorder at the beginning of the pandemic, though the memories that bothered me were from many years earlier. For several months it felt like the past was percolating through the present, shapeshifting the world. I had been to Afghanistan, Syria, and Iraq, and there were times I thought I was going to die or I felt undone by stories of genocide, loss, and rape.

The experiences made me feel lonely and disconnected, but I never lived the unreality of trauma until the pandemic. The empty streets, the body trucks, the isolation—they must have made my nervous system feel trapped, as if back in a war zone.

We're not supposed to constantly live in a threatened state. We're supposed to be able to go into these states when needed, and come out when the threat is over. PTSD can be understood as a disorder in which the shift into a defensive state doesn't extinguish, it doesn't turn off, and you get stuck there. And you live with this altered sense of time and space—what some people call trauma time—in which the sexual assault or the war is still happening, it's not over. And you keep responding to threats in the here and now, because you experience cues that are associated strongly enough with the trauma that they activate the action systems of defense against it.

And when one is in a dissociated state, there are alterations to how you experience the present situation, of time and space, of identity, of memory. I remember how the noise of helicopters didn't cease, how they were everywhere those days, swooping low in neighborhoods, patrolling protests in Brooklyn. My apartment walls were too thin and the windows too old. Days passed and the noise didn't stop. I remember wanting to cover my head from the mortars that weren't there. I remember sitting on my couch, staring at the wall, feeling afraid. That was when the wall started to thin, the ceiling opened to the sky, and it felt as if the wind and sand were pelting my face. I was looking again through the lens of a telescope and seeing the Islamic State flag in the pale sky.

On another day, a limp summer day in the Hudson Valley, I walked on a trail through tall grass. The grass was blowing and bending. I looked up at the quiet oak trees. I felt like I was in Syria again, when the Americans told us we had to run from snipers. That was before we saw the dead body in the ruined village.

The experiences were disorienting, but I never doubted the reality of them because they fit easily into a long tradition of war writing—the hallucinatory texts of Michael Herr, Tim O'Brien, Kurt Vonnegut, Brian Turner. "War is a surrealistic experience," O'Brien told an early biographer. "I see myself as a realist in the strictest sense. That is to say, our daydreams are real; our fantasies are real."

When I talked to victims of sexual violence, they described similar moments, but I didn't immediately connect these kinds of experiences to any larger storytelling tradition. (And, of course, rape survivors' stories aren't generally treated as heroic or sites of transcendence.) I thought instead about how this kind of storytelling leaves women trapped in legal questions of believability and trustworthiness.

But rape and sexual assault can also be experienced as "unreality," or what one victim called the "sexual surreal." Faces can morph, or victims might feel the weight of invisible hands on their backs. Victims might see their bodies as distorted or no longer human. They've reported experiences of depersonalization and derealization, indicating a feeling of unreality or detachment from the world and the self—a lack of familiarity. And changes in perception: a hand shrinks, a mouth grows large. A sound coming from a few feet away might be perceived as coming from a great distance.

In one study, victims of childhood sexual abuse were asked to write narratives about their trauma. And they wrote incoherent and confusing stories: switching between past and present, adulthood and childhood. They struggled to find words and formulate sentences to describe experiences of dissociation. They switched pronouns. They described fragments of experiences in a chaotic manner, with incomplete or long sentences that were hard to follow. Punctuation disappeared. Sentences were left alone and suspended. The texts included symbols.

It's riskier for victims of sexual trauma to narrate these

stories because "believability" has been the primary burden of their telling, in a way that is less true for war stories, torture, natural disasters, or other experiences of suffering.

Even though women are more likely than men to suffer from trauma, the history of psychological suffering is typically told as a straight line from shell shock in the First World War to PTSD in the wake of Vietnam. And, as the authors of *Gender and Trauma Since 1900* have written: "Women are often erased entirely from this master narrative."

Consider this journal entry from 1889 by explorer David Livingstone, who recorded his numb and dreamlike experience of tonic immobility while being attacked by a lion:

> It caused a sort of dreaminess, in which there was no sense of pain or feeling of terror, though quite conscious of all that was happening. It was like what patients partially under the influence of chloroform describe, who see all the operation, but feel not the knife. This singular condition was not the result of any mental process. The shake annihilated fear, and allowed no sense of horror in looking around at the beast. This peculiar state is probably produced in all animals killed by carnivora; and if so, it is a merciful provision by our benevolent Creator for lessening the pain of death.

What if this experience happened, but instead of a lion it was a rapist? Would you ever be able to explain the experience of "dreaminess" to a police officer, a prosecutor, or a jury? Would you tell them there was no terror and no pain? You probably wouldn't. It would feel like a risk—you wouldn't want to sound insensible.

. . .

Sometimes during a rape, or a sexual assault, a person might feel something more taboo than nothing: pleasure in the body. There are orgasms without joy and erections without desire. "It's difficult to accept, but it's a reality," French psychologist Coraline Hingray told me. "It's just a physiological reaction. Of course, most don't feel anything because they are numb or they dissociate. But sometimes there could be some lubrication or pleasure."

"I orgasmed when he did it," a woman in her twenties told me, "and so I've never wanted to talk about it. I always think maybe it wasn't rape."

"I hate myself for it," said another. "It's kept me quiet."

Hingray thinks society needs a different word for undesired orgasms that happen in the midst of sexual violence. When she talks to her patients—both men and women—she uses the word "orgast": a physiological reaction to physical stimulation without desire.

In 2019, the psychologist Meredith Chivers exposed men and women to sexually explicit images and measured physiological signs of arousal as well as subjective feelings of desire. The images included nude bodies, heterosexual and homosexual sex, as well as bonobo sex. The men responded predictably to images that matched their sexual orientation, while the women in the study didn't. The women were physiologically aroused by all the images, even the bonobos having sex. But it didn't mean that this physical arousal was connected to desire. The women didn't desire to have sex with the people or animals they saw, despite their bodies' responses. In a similar study from 2011, the authors found that their female participants "exhibited genital responses to narratives involving sexual assault and extreme violence, which they nevertheless described as very unpleasant."

When Hingray proposed the topic of "orgast" at a conference, it was rejected. "No one wanted to discuss it," she said. "But it is quite frequent, especially if you live with lots of sexual assault or if you lived with it during your childhood."

I remember when a professor read Yeats's poem "Leda and the Swan": "How can those terrified vague fingers push / The feathered glory from her loosening thighs?"

How he read it with delight, circling a wooden school chair like a bird of prey.

"Raptor" has its root in the Latin for *rapere*—seizing, taking, tearing away, raping. "Raptor" is the agent noun, the plunderer, the ravisher. "Rapt" (and later "rapture") by the Middle Ages came to refer to sexual and spiritual ecstasy as well as to rape. And religious scholar Julie B. Miller writes that the "spiritual notion of rapture is highly informed by the sexually violent connotations of rape."

Women saints in the medieval period wrote extensively about encounters with God in imagery that is filled with wounding and agony, tangled with erotic delight.

The thirteenth-century Christian mystic Mechthild of Magdeburg was amazed by "the violent force of love." In the fifteenth century, Catherine of Genoa wrote that "rays" of God's love are always "hungrily seeking to penetrate" humanity and, if given the chance, will penetrate "as deep as hell." God sent Catherine of Genoa a ray of his love "so burning and deep that it was an agony to sustain. . . . The soul cried out, sighed deeply, and in its transformation, was taken out of itself."

In the sixteenth century, Teresa of Ávila often attempted to resist the assaults, but ultimately knew she couldn't fight God and accepted it, because it was going to happen anyway. The women were living in patriarchal worlds and these responses were a negotiation with their circumstances; sometimes the only avenue to power was through an attempt to encounter God, often through violence and wounds.

In Bernini's sculpture of Saint Teresa of Ávila in Rome, she appears to be orgasming in ecstasy as an angel prepares to impale her with God's love in the form of a golden spear.

"When he drew it out," Saint Teresa wrote, "I thought he was carrying off with him the deepest part of me; and he left me all on fire with great love of God. The pain was so great that it made me moan."

In other words, rape and ecstasy were always circling each other.

In the front seat of a car, in a wooded area of rural South Carolina, a woman was choked and raped, and she ascended to a light where she was warm, safe, and whole, and separate from her body.

Another was sexually assaulted in a bathroom, then ascended into a light-filled world and danced with Michael Jackson on a cloud.

Reports of near-death experiences, or NDEs, often involve tunnels and lights and figures. Some people talk of visiting new worlds, have a feeling that time is altered, or a sense of harmony with the environment, and some relive past events, like a life review. Sometimes such near-death experiences are reported by victims of sexual violence.

The neuroscientist Charlotte Martial is one of the world's leading experts on NDEs and part of a team at the Coma Science Group who hypothesized that tonic immobility is the evolutionary origin of near-death experiences. Both are triggered by life-threatening events and ease emotional distress. And what made tonic immobility evolve into NDEs? "Our acquisition of language transformed these perceptions into rich and complex stories. Like the impression that they are leaving their body," Martial told me, "or seeing a very bright light, or a tunnel. Or when they meet entities or alien beings, people we know or strangers."

Near-death experiences are typically associated with positive emotion. So the hypothesis here is that when humans are in a very distressing situation, they will create a new reality in their minds to ease their suffering.

The International Association for Near-Death Studies keeps their own database of NDEs and out-of-body experiences, and I found dozens related to sexual violence.

Anonymous, 7/8/24:

The first out-of-body experience that I had was when I was 18 and a man attacked me and violently raped me threatening to strangle me. He had thrown me into the back of his van. I was sure I was going to die. I did not scream or move. I just lay rigid and then I found myself up near the roof of the van looking down on us both. When he stopped, I went back into my body.

Being raped—and not crying out—had a profound effect on me and about a year later I tried to kill myself. I was taken in a coma to hospital and was given a stomach pump etc. Then I was put in a private room in a psychiatric clinic with a nurse on guard. When I came round and opened my eyes and saw her and realized where I was, I left my body for a second time and again hovered above in the corner of the room. There was no strong, "wonderful" feeling about this, nor any fear of death. I simply felt safe, "removed," out of reach. They couldn't do anything to me.

In October 2010, a college student wrote that she woke up at three in the morning to find her boyfriend raping her with his hands around her neck. "I just slid out of my body," she wrote. "I was hovering at the ceiling, totally detached emotionally from my body. I watched him continue to rape and abuse my body without much emotion. I felt wonderful with no pain or negative emotions. It was as if every cell in my body was in ecstasy."

She added, "I was terrified of explaining this whole experience to police. I couldn't imagine what I would say."

In December 2012, another woman reported, "I awoke and found a male assailant beside my bed, and unfortunately I did not have my glasses on. When I sat up, the assailant put his hands around my throat, and as I struggled, his grip became harder until I passed out." When she opened her eyes, she saw herself on the bed and the assailant on top of her. She was watching it all from above the bathroom door. A few moments later she was surrounded by a burst of light. "All pain and paralyzing fear disappeared," she wrote. And she entered a tunnel of light, and she had no hands and no body.

She added, "I couldn't disclose this event to anyone because I felt I would have been placed in an institution."

While thinking about this topic, I came across Kathryn Harrison's description of violence in her 1997 memoir, *The Kiss*.

The sight of him naked: at that point I fall completely asleep. I arrive at the state promised by the narcotic kiss in the airport. In years to come, I won't be able to remember one instance of our lying together. I'll have a composite, generic memory. I'll know that he was always on top and that I always lay still, as still as if I had, in truth, fallen from a great height. . . . No matter how hard I try, pushing myself to inhabit my past, I'll recoil from what will always seem impossible.

When I read this paragraph for the first time, I thought it was perfect, at least as a way to write about something so horrible. It was showing us the traumatic mind at work, rather than trying to get around it. We see the mind in an act of escape.

"But, as a reader, as a lover of stories, I must confess I'm disappointed," writer David McGlynn wrote of this same scene in *Bending Genre: Essays on Creative Nonfiction*. "It's not that I want a graphic sex scene between a middle-aged father and his teenage daughter, but I'm nevertheless bored by the author's 'composite, generic memories.' "

Harrison's lack of sensation is the memory. Numb and empty; out of body, out of the scene. The recoiling is not so much "self-conscious," as McGlynn writes, but loyal to her response.

If she doesn't want to remember her body at that moment, is it really that important for the pleasure of the reader? McGlynn suggests Harrison embrace magical realism, something more along the lines of Tim O'Brien's *The Things They Carried*, which not only embraced the surreal nature of experience but mixed fact with the author's fantasy to tell a more compelling story. O'Brien called this "story-truth," which is different from "happening-truth," a term he used to describe the actual experience lived by authors or their characters.

Were the stakes different for stories of sexual violence? Stories of frozen women are often quiet stories, not necessarily interesting stories. The princess wakes up from a hundred-year sleep with two suckling babies. With no memory of life as she slept, what story is there to tell?

There hasn't been much time to understand how to tell these stories. It's only in the last fifty years or so that women's stories of sexual harm have mattered enough to be recorded and read about. What did women do when their stories were too dangerous, counterintuitive, or strange? In *The Heroine with 1001 Faces*, Maria Tatar mentions a British fairy tale called "Mr. Fox," and in the tale the heroine tells a story of violence by calling it a dream. The "dream story" protects her from being silenced in the telling, but also gives her a medium for telling her stories with surreal and symbolic elements of narrative.

I learned that in the nineteenth century, violated women told their stories through the stories of vivisected animals. Most anti-vivisectionists were women. "It was not simply for reasons of humanity," historian Coral Lansbury wrote in *The Old Brown Dog: Women, Workers, and Vivisection in Edwardian England*, "but because the vivisected animal stood for vivisected women: the women strapped to the gynecologist's table, the women strapped and bound in the pornographic fiction of the period."

The rise of medical technology and knowledge created new terrors for women. In the 1860s, with the passage of the Contagious Disease Acts in the United Kingdom, women were being taken off the streets and forcibly inspected with speculums. In 1870, a doctor named J. J. Wilkinson published testimonies of these women, where he described the "forcing open of women's bodies with large glass instruments or with large expanding steel instruments" and women enduring "long minutes of torture" and "corresponding destruction afterward." He wrote of "women thus opened alive." He wrote of a violated "menstruating girl" to whom "the doctor said that if she did not comply, he would declare her diseased, and send her to the Lock Hospital." He observed that many women "walking home after it, stooped, and wept as they walked, with flushed faces, and a look of pain, which no woman who has ever suffered such pain can mistake."

At the same time, many women were undergoing forced surgeries without the use of anesthetic, including having their healthy ovaries removed. Elizabeth Blackwell, the first woman to receive an American medical degree, called ovarian removal "the castration of women," and some gynecological textbooks at the time called it "spaying." In 1886, one in every 250 women had the procedure, and in France alone there were at least 500,000 "spayed" women.

The animal rights activist Anna Kingsford used her dreams of tortured animals to express her concerns about women. "I went in my sleep last night from one torture-chamber to another in the underground vaults of a vivisector's laboratory, and in all were men at work lacerating, dissecting, and burning the living flesh of their victims. But these were no longer mere horses or dogs or rabbits; for in each I saw a human shape."

When anti-vivisectionist Frances Cobbe lectured on the cruel experiments conducted by men on dogs, the women in her audience openly sobbed, expressing what Coral Lansbury called a "subterranean horror." Lansbury saw it everywhere. When Elizabeth Blackwell denounced the way women were treated, she never directly described the horror she observed, but spoke of it indirectly, using animals as surrogates for women's experiences of horror.

To make her point, Lansbury quotes Elizabeth Browning's nineteenth-century novel *Aurora Leigh*: "The works of women are symbolical." And when the symbolic language is drawn from vivisected animals, Lansbury says, the message is even more "potent" as it is "drawn from a muffled context of reticence and silence."

Is this why the first animal shelter was built in 1869—almost one hundred years before the first shelter for battered women?

———

For ten years Stacie—the woman without memories of childhood—worked with Jim Helling, a therapist in western Massachusetts who specializes in dissociative disorders. "I like to think about dissociation as a gift evolution gave us," Helling told me over the phone, "so that we can perform a kind of magic to save ourselves when there's no other recourse."

Helling liked to work with clients through their own symbolic storytelling. And clients will come to his office, he said, to share their dreams of imprisonment.

One was a woman with severe anorexia who dreamed of enjoying herself at summer camp until she realized everyone had perfect bodies and exercised endlessly, and those who were less than perfect began to disappear from camp. They were being watched and evaluated, and no one was allowed to leave. It wasn't summer camp, but a concentration camp, and the campers existed in a state of living death. The dream came again and again. She tried to escape the camp but was caught and brought back. "The capacity to dream was an articulation," he said, and "it was a frightful image of what she was struggling with internally." Starving herself wasn't working to keep herself safe, and over time she let this defense of hers grow weak.

Another client dreamed about a cave full of hidden jewels that were guarded by a large dragon. The dragon wasn't the danger; he was just responsible for preserving the jewels. "So that dragon deserves gratitude and respect and honor for its role, and you can't fault the dragon for not recognizing when it's okay to let someone pass to have access—its job was to preserve at all costs."

"The clients dreamed of Dis," Helling said. In *Dante's Inferno*, Dis is Lucifer, God's most beautiful, renegade angel who rules over a frozen lake of traitors. *Dis*avowal, *dis*connection, *dis*ease, even *dis*aster, which means to become separated from your stars. Dis is the personification of the dark side of our defenses, he explained—their imprisoning powers.

Helling was drawing from the work of Donald Kalshed, a Jungian psychologist who believed traumatized people often had dreams about animals and nature, or figures associated with protection. So while dissociation makes life possible and serves a protective function, "it sequesters part of ourselves in a kind of suspended animation until conditions are favorable for that to reemerge."

He explained it like this: If you get attacked by a lion or a bear and it's tearing your body apart, blood is withdrawn from the periphery of your body. You'll give up an arm, you'll give up a leg. This is what keeps you alive. So you will protect the center—you will give up all the nonessentials, and protect and preserve what sustains life. Helling believes there's a very similar mechanism at work in our psyche. The person who's being sexually assaulted or otherwise attacked has this experience of rising out of their body and heading to the ceiling—this is not just to protect them, he explained: "It moves something away. What it moves away is the thing that's most precious, the thing that's most worthy of protecting. But sometimes people will put something someplace where they can't find it again on their own without help."

One spring I drove to the small town of Weyers Cave, in the Shenandoah Valley, on the edge of the Blue Ridge Mountains in Virginia, to visit a local police academy. The building was modern, with carpeted floors and windows that looked out at chestnut and oak forests. I was here to attend a training taught by Nancy Oglesby, a retired prosecutor with a birdlike frame and ethereal white hair, and Mike Milnor, a retired police chief with a shaved head and a goatee, aimed at helping cops and prosecutors understand the way trauma affects storytelling.

One of the most common problems facing prosecutors in sexual-assault cases is the tendency of defense lawyers to portray the normal behavior of women, both during and after their experiences, as "unusual" or "inconsistent." Oglesby and Milnor wanted to help people see the world the way the victim was seeing it.

In the room were police deputies, campus police officers, members of special-victims units, detectives, victim advocates, social workers, sexual-assault-hotline workers, CIA agents. A few off-duty cops wore Glocks on their hips. Occasionally cadets marched in unison down the hallways.

Oglesby and Milnor talked to them about how traumatic events are more difficult to recount in a linear manner; how it will be harder to answer those who-what-where-why questions. Instead, a victim's ability to explain the event is going to be more tied to sensory perceptions as opposed to some kind of narrative. Milnor wanted to teach the cops how to let victims tell their own stories. Sensory stories, weird stories, stories that made no sense. To let them tell stories through their bodies, through what the body was feeling, and images that seemed like nothing but mental detritus. Whatever it was, if they remembered it, write it down. Each trauma response might be accompanied by very different sensations.

But police too often followed an interrogation technique that taught them to assume that when a statement wasn't detailed, or if there were gaps or inconsistencies in the account, the person was lying.

"When there were a lot of 'I don't knows,' 'I don't remembers' in sexual-assault statements, that created proof problems," Nancy Oglesby told me. There was once a case she had decided not to pursue because she couldn't make sense of different memories in the story: A young woman was raped in a dorm room, and her roommate was knocking on the door and yelling, trying to get in. The suspect remembered this and described the knocking and yelling exactly as it happened. The victim said no one knocked on the door. Why wouldn't the victim have that same memory?

Now Oglesby knows that sensory perceptions will be different depending on trauma responses. And some responses change what people pay attention to and thus what sort of memories they have of an experience. A victim who enters a state of tonic immobility, for example, might have rigid muscles or trembling limbs or might feel extremely cold. But if she dissociated at the same time, she won't remember those details because she will have had no awareness of what was going on in her body at the time. A victim may find herself focused on details that investigators find irrelevant but that her brain processes as important for survival, whether it's the color of a wall or a song playing down the hall or the patterns of veins in a leaf on a plant a few feet away. In dark rooms, attention might drift to digital clocks or mirrors. It's why a victim might not know the color of the shirt her attacker was wearing or even whether he wore a condom. It's also not unusual for survivors to have vivid memories about the beginning of a sexual assault when the initial burst of stress hormones was released.

If a victim takes a case to trial, the defense is going to try to argue that their memories of "irrelevant things," their lack of memories about "relevant" details, and the lack of chronology in telling mean the victim is being deceitful. "We try to flip that," Oglesby said. "Okay, if they're experiencing one of these neurobiological responses, they're not going to be able to give you a play-by-play of what happened during the assault— which traditionally is how we looked at the credibility of a victim statement."

Early in his career, Milnor said behaviors like freezing and tonic immobility were the most difficult to understand. There was one woman who told him she couldn't move her legs. And another who said she tried to scream but nothing came out. Why wouldn't she scream if there were people nearby? Then he was tasked with death notifications, and the first time he knocked on a door it was to tell a family their son had died in a car accident.

"The wife just went completely immobile on me," he said. "She went catatonic. Her husband and I literally set her down on the sofa like a robot. It was like she was just gone, but her eyes were still open."

Now Milnor knows that when a woman says she "froze," it could mean many things.

"I'll say, 'Well, can you tell me more about that? Can you tell me what sensations you can remember feeling? Do you remember how things sounded? Are there any smells?' I would just go through the five senses," he told me. It's these physiological details and feelings and sensations that Milnor encourages people to look for in their investigations.

Milnor dimmed the lights, and a projector hummed to life. On the screen, he showed us pages from an investigator's notebook, where the victim talked for five hours, and the detective wrote everything down without interruption. The notes resembled a map with archipelagoes of words and oceans of empty space in between, and dozens of arrows connected the islands to form a single story. "This is how it will look," he said.

Milnor admitted that he'd made some mistakes with sexual-assault victims, that he was guilty of thinking that some women's statements were too outlandish to be true. He had messed up, and knew all the cops in the room had messed up too.

"How many of you remember," Milnor said at one point, "having a victim do something where you just kind of tilted your head and thought, Wait, that didn't make any sense?"

Many nodded and shifted in their seats.

"Remember how many times we judged a victim because we didn't understand their behavior? Maybe they were texting their abuser the day after the assault and saying, 'Hey, did you have a good time?'"

More nodding.

Milnor assured the group that he, too, had done all that. He said the way he once responded to victims still keeps him up at night. "Now I teach from my mistakes," he said.

Anne Munch is an attorney in Colorado who worked on sexual-assault cases for thirty years. "We have so many double standards around victim behavior," she told me. "We have so many excuses around offender behavior. But it starts with law enforcement. I tell police, 'Your response to victims will make or break the case, and you might make or break the person.'"

Munch told me about a police report she received early in her career. A woman in her twenties met friends at a bar and drank too much. The woman called a cab to go home, and the driver took her to a remote location, parked the car, got into the back seat, and raped her. When he finished, he got back in the driver's seat and took her home. She paid the fare, and he left.

Munch thought there had to be more to the story, so she met the victim for another interview. She asked open-ended questions that would give the woman a sense of control, and she tried to unlock memories by asking about senses. The woman told her that when the driver got in the back of the cab, it became clear that the rape would happen, so she turned her head and stared at the cab door until it was over. The victim described the material on the door in striking detail—a gray vinyl with a stitched pattern like an ellipsis, a chrome handle with exactly eight small indentations from the bottom to the top.

Munch had just come out of the child-sex-abuse unit and knew a lot about children and dissociation. She recognized it when she heard it. "The woman was describing a classic dissociative response," Munch said. "Her normal coping mechanisms are overwhelmed. What's happening is too big, too ugly, too much." Munch sent her investigator to the cab company with a search warrant, and everything was exactly the way the victim had described it. Munch told the defense that she was going to recommend a trauma expert to speak at the trial. "If this sex is so great and consensual, then why is she turning her head and memorizing the inside of the taxicab?" she recalled saying. The driver pleaded guilty, which saved the woman from going to trial.

Later, I bought copies of *The Investigator Anthology* and *A Field Guide to the Reid Technique,* the manuals that Milnor and Oglesby said outlined the gold standard of police interrogation, known as the Reid technique. The anthology was particularly enormous, with a forest-green cover. They were both filled with rape myths.

I went through each manual and annotated it with Milnor's responses from the training.

The manuals state that "an assault that is reported immediately is more likely to be truthful" (not true—sexual assaults are rarely reported immediately) and that cops should "look for inconsistencies in the victim's statement about the suspect and the assault," because they were signs of deception (not true). It instructed police to watch out for "illogical behavior during the assault." (Illogical behavior can be a normal response to trauma.)

A section called "Establishing the Truthfulness of a Sexual Assault Victim" explains why a sexual-assault victim would lie. (Lying is extremely rare.) This includes "a desire for attention," "a way to cover up unfaithfulness," "a fear of pregnancy or STD," "a desire for revenge, or because of a custody battle or divorce." (All sexist.) The manual instructs that a "victim should be evaluated with respect to a histrionic or borderline personality disorder. Histrionic females are typically attractive and fashion conscious." ("So, if your victim is good-looking and she's got a nice dress on, she has three strikes against her?" Milnor said.)

"When a victim is relaying a free-flowing account of the incident be aware of the spontaneous phrase: I can't remember what happened then." (Gaps in memory are normal.)

"The victim who one minute is answering questions in total control and then breaks into a crying spell and wipes dry eyes with a tissue, and within a few seconds is able to return to the interview fully composed may be feigning distress." (Changes in composure are normal.)

"If you ask the victim, 'Why do you think that man did this thing?' a truthful victim will say he has to be sick or a pervert. The deceptive answer is 'I don't know' or 'I really haven't thought about it.'" (Neither one of these responses relates to truth or deception.)

———

When Stacie was eighteen, her mom finally decided to leave her abusive husband. He threatened to kill them if they left, but they did it anyway. It took months to plan. One day, after they escaped, they decided to go back to the house to get some important mail. Her mom's car was stopped and running by the curb while Stacie ran to the mailbox. They thought he was at work, but he wasn't. Stacie's stepdad came charging out. She bolted for the car, and made it inside, but he was fast. He had a grip on her leg and was trying to pull her out through the window while Stacie's mom was pulling her in. He pulled so hard the door handle broke. That's a memory she holds but does not feel. She was too dissociated to have access to the emotions.

Her therapist thought it would be important for her to feel the memory.

They visited the memory from Stacie's perspective first, when she was inside the car, being pulled by her mom and her stepdad. She felt nothing. Instead, she went back into the memory from the perspective of her neighbor. She watched what was happening to this girl, who happened to be herself—Stacie—and this time she felt something: She felt horribly afraid for that girl. As a neighbor, she could see, objectively, how terrible it all was. But she had to inhabit a different body, a different perspective, to be able to feel any emotional connection to her own experience of fear and pain.

Jim Helling, the therapist who worked with Stacie, said many Jungians think of dissociation as "a little bit of a Sleeping Beauty story." Our access to the dissociated material, to the Sleeping Beauty, is prevented by the briars. "In the old story," he explained, "before it was called 'Sleeping Beauty,' it was called 'Briar Rose,' because around the castle where the young woman sleeps after she pricks her finger on the spindle (the traumatic disruption) is this incredibly thick, impenetrable rose vine with huge thorns. And the hero has to find his way through the briars to reach the young woman and reanimate her and bring her back to life with a kiss." He paused and then added, "It's a bit of a sexist story. We probably need a new one."

Sometimes Stacie had to find her way back to her body again. She had to notice when she experienced pain, because she hadn't felt pain in a long time. She had to start recognizing what her body was feeling, and sometimes therapy meant she was just sitting in a room, feeling her body and paying attention to it. She had felt no pain for many years, and now, suddenly, she felt a lot of pain: in her chest she felt tightness, in her stomach she felt an ache. She was literally teaching herself to feel because she was so disconnected from her body. Then, slowly, she would try to name the sensations. It had been easy for her to hurt herself and not recognize it. She found she needed to take notes about accidents: *I ran into the table and hit my knee today*. If she knew about the pain, she would be able to help her body. Once she took care of the parts that hurt, usually that meant she was able to recognize pain somewhere else. She had leg pain and knee pain; she had pain in her wrist and chest and in her stomach. Was the pain always there? Had she just dissociated so severely from her body that she didn't feel it? She knew that soldiers fighting in combat didn't get hungry. They didn't sleep. They didn't feel the urge to drink or defecate or urinate. Everything was shut down so that all their energy and attention could go into fighting, which meant staying alive. But once there was a break, the soldier might be overcome with the pain and hunger and thirst. Stacie had been living life as stressed as a combat soldier.

For a long time she didn't feel hunger either, and it took years of working with her body to feel it again. When she journals to try to make sense of things, she knows she's done if she feels the ache of hunger.

I thought of my own dissociations and the desire to feel again. I thought of the time I went to see friends after a reporting trip to a drug market in Philadelphia. How I had watched an addicted woman have a psychotic break and stab her friend in the neck with a broken crack pipe. I ran over to help the woman, her eyes unblinking, perfectly round. She wouldn't go to the hospital because she was too high on heroin.

"That's what you get for trying to be a good person," she kept saying. The other woman was her friend and she had been helping her with something. I gave her money for a cab to go to the hospital even though I knew she wasn't going to go. She was too scared of getting in trouble for the drugs. So she walked off, white as a ghost. I took the train home and went straight to a dinner party. I was there but not really there. My friends were laughing and applying makeup samples. I didn't think I heard anything they said. I was so far away, still with the woman in Philadelphia, watching the blood spurt out of her neck.

For my own memories I was asked to go back and rescript them. My trauma specialist was a woman with short hair and highlights wearing a purple cardigan and oversize jewelry. I'd never heard of EMDR (eye movement desensitization and reprocessing), but I was willing to try it. EMDR activates both brain hemispheres in order to link emotion to experience. When the right brain gets stimulated, many of the raw emotions that were stored but unreachable become available. By activating the left hemisphere you can link new emotions to memories by reimagining the experience.

I was supposed to recall a difficult memory to send my brain into a panic, and then add a new ending, or retell the story to make it less threatening.

I started with the dead body, which I saw in Syria. I decided on this because it was recent and concrete. It wasn't complicated. No one wants to see a dead body.

I was asked to reimagine the memory either by replacing a negative belief with a positive one, or by rewriting the scenes in the memory itself. The idea was this: If I could reimagine a memory, I would no longer feel overwhelmed by it.

"What's the point?" I asked the therapist. "I'll know the new memory isn't real, right?"

The fact of my memory being real or not mattered to me. It seemed impossible that we were actually going to revise a memory, but I pushed against even the possibility of it. I hated what I had experienced, but I also valued it. I would rather carry the sad truths that I had sought out and that I had witnessed than be free of them.

But she assured me we weren't tricking our minds, only the nervous system. "Our nervous systems don't know the difference between fact and fiction," she told me. And I found this comforting. It meant I could hold on to real memories while also finding refuge in imagined ones. I would still have the memories, but I could link them to new emotions. That way I couldn't be overwhelmed by them. They were just inert.

"Imagine everything you should have said," she told me, "or that you'd like to say now." I entered the memory like a video-game character, and started tinkering. You can do whatever you want, she told me, no limits.

I didn't know what to do about the dead man. He was an Islamic State soldier and I tried to imagine his life before he'd become radicalized. I wondered about his family. I could see his underwear, which was blue, and made me see him as someone's child. There was not much to revise, but sitting with the memory and imagining him as fully human helped me look at the memory and experience it, which I had never done, because I was too quick to look away. "In these situations," the therapist said, " 'I survived' is sometimes the only good thing to come out of a situation. The simple fact of being alive."

The periods that followed sessions were difficult. I slept through whole days. I was nauseated and ate only because I knew I should. A deep immobilizing depression overcame me and then quickly let me go. It was as if my body needed to feel these emotions one last time before I was free of them. These were the emotions my brain had cut off to protect me and now they were rushing back in.

The memories were still there, but they were different. Far away, out of reach. Snuffed of heartbreak, drained of terror. I kept editing, revisiting, dampening memories. I saw everything in reverse, the blood returning to the body of the soldier killed in the field by the American boy who knew too little about his trigger. The snarled lips relaxed back over his teeth and his mouth closed. I saw the sweat rise back up to his hair. I saw his tilted body return to his feet, saw the two men back away from each other, back into the tall grass, back into their lives. We were nearby, running from snipers.

The dragon guarded the precious jewels, and the birds sang back to me. Christ came down from the crucifix. How far back could I go? As far back as my mother had gone to inhabit past lives, using an imagined past to cope with the present? It didn't seem so different.

"Re-vision," writes Adrienne Rich, "the act of looking back, of seeing with fresh eyes, of entering an old text from a new critical direction . . . is an act of survival."

When I saw my friends again, they said, "You seem here." And I had the same question as so many women I talked to had asked themselves: Well, if I'm here, then where had I been?

Fear and Trembling

I KNEW THE BEAVERS WERE NEARBY BECAUSE I COULD SMELL them. A dense odor fragrant with mineral and pine. I saw the steam rise from the little snow-covered chimney at the top of their lodge. I was at a friend's house, and we'd been out playing but lost track of each other, and I didn't care now, because I had found the beavers. I could dive into the river and stick my head inside their den to see them. It's what I wanted to do. I imagined the warmth of their bodies, the sawdust beds, the little glowing eyes. The mud burped and sucked at my bare feet as I walked into the river.

It was spring, and most of the snow had melted, but there were still patches along the river and on top of the spruce trees. When I plunged beneath the surface, I couldn't see anything but shades of green and brown. I dove twice into the murky deep, then gave up. On the way back to my friend's house I started shivering, and at first the tremors were small and not uncomfortable, but they grew and became spastic and my body started to hurt. My teeth clacked. If someone had walked by they might have thought I was dancing. I could no longer move my fingers. I knew what was happening to me, and that I had been careless, and I kept walking, and as I walked I stopped for a moment because I heard the beavers laughing at me. I so badly wanted to go back to them but I knew I shouldn't. I knew I was on the edge of life and death, becoming hypothermic, an in-between place that was strange but was also keeping me alive. The convulsions were uncomfortable but I understood them as a way to keep me warm.

When I peeled off my socks, I found flaccid colorless feet with blue toes. I massaged the flesh and warmth brought with it a violent stinging, a kind of tortured renewal.

While freezing deadens, it also offers a chance for salvation. Maybe that's why I was collecting stories of frozen women coming back to life. I had become obsessed with the image of the frozen women, seeing a reflection of myself again and again in these lifeless bodies, searching for meaning, not yet understanding the lifesaving use of a body in repose. It started when my husband's mother went into sudden cardiac arrest and, to save her, they cooled her down by about eight degrees. The cold kept her safe. The colder the body, the less oxygen the brain needs to function. Blood flow slows, the heart barely beats, and we become like animals in hibernation, existing in a state of suspension between life and death.

From a 1999 story, "Woman 'frozen' in lake brought back to life," in *The Guardian*:

Anna Bågenholm, 29, a trainee surgeon, was skiing off-piste, near Narvik, in northern Norway, when she fell through a frozen river and became trapped under the ice for 40 minutes. As colleagues struggled to rescue her from beneath the ice, her body temperature gradually dropped and her vital organs shut down. Her temperature had fallen more than 23 degrees below normal. No one is known to have lived after becoming so cold before. The previous survival record was held by a child whose temperature fell to 14.4 C.

"Frozen Ordeal Has Happy Ending," read a headline from a 1980 issue of Minnesota's *Thirteen Towns*:

> Jean was driving home from visiting a friend when the family car skidded on ice and became trapped in a snowbank. She sought shelter from the 22 below zero temperatures.... She headed for Wally Nelson's home two miles from the marooned car. She didn't make it. She collapsed and lay in the snow for six hours. She was found by Nelson at 7 a.m. as he headed for work at the Fosston Locker Plant.

He knew her face. She was glittering in the sunlight, about fifteen feet from the door. She had tumbled and crawled—he saw the tracks in the snow

She was solid with eyes frozen open and no movable joints. He was sure she was dead until he saw some bubbles in her nose. The rancher tried loading Jean's body into the cab of his truck. Jean was too stiff to fit in the cab, so he had to diagonally load her into the back seat of a car that belonged to the woman he'd brought home from the bar the night before.

Jean's body temperature was 80.6°F, pulse twelve beats per minute. The doctors broke needles on her frozen skin. They didn't have much hope. They'd never had a frozen girl show up like this. George Sather was the physician. "Just like a piece of meat out of a deep freeze," he told the media. They figured she was mostly dead but tried to thaw her anyway with heating pads and moist cloths. She started to wake up in spasms—legs kicking, arms shaking, quivering muscles. After forty-nine days in the hospital, she walked out completely resurrected.

For years I had chronic pain in my right hip flexor and eventually learned my hip bone was out of place, twisted and frozen that way. The first time I went to have the hip unstuck, in 2018, the physical therapist yanked it back into place and sent me home. That night, my right torso erupted into contractions so painful I was sobbing, could not walk, and needed muscle relaxants to stop the spasms.

After that, the pain was all over my body, and it moved around from one part to another. My hip kept contracting back into its stuck place, and I kept having to go back and have it adjusted. One physical therapist told me it looked like I was holding my body in a braced position as if ready for some sort of an attack. Another noticed that I was stiff only on the right side of the body. She told me, "Like it's dead or something."

Another called it "space ice cream."

I was in pain but didn't know what was wrong. I spent the next year going from one doctor to the next.

"Well, nothing is wrong with you," the doctor at Mount Sinai said.

I was simply stiff. Fear and stress had hardened my muscles, twisting bones and ligaments out of place. Even after being loosened, the muscles returned to their wooden state.

Finally I found a woman who was able to look closely at my body and help me. She noticed I held my body in a kind of wounded limp. She was the kind of therapist who specialized in fear-stiffened bodies, stuck bodies. Bodies dried out like space ice cream.

The first thing she did was pick up my leg and shake it. The table rocked. She was always rocking women's bodies on tables, letting them loosely flop.

"Moving the body," she told me, "tells the body that you're safe."

I noticed that some part of my body was always trying to move—but only at night. I chomped through a mouth guard and swallowed plastic. I kicked and scratched. A couple of times I pulled out my eyelashes. Night was a frenzy of activity. I often woke up covered in tiny scratches, all from my own nails.

As she stretched and massaged and released muscle and fascia, I trembled and shivered. My body was a symphony of spasms: quads, back, shoulders, neck, arms. Sometimes the twitches felt like a chorus; like little parts of me were waking up, moving wildly—the opposite of frozen.

One of her clients refused to be rocked. She couldn't take it. She wasn't ready. The client was so disconnected from her own body that she couldn't feel the table and she was worried she was going to fall to the ground.

The pain moved around my body like an elusive animal. I felt haunted by it. It moved to my wrist and forearm. Back to my jaw, my neck. She hunted the pain. I was given patches to stick on my muscles "to help me remember my body." They smelled of camphor.

One day, while she worked my body, I remembered having the uncomfortable desire to thrash, almost like I wanted to escape the room and run. I tried to keep still, but I couldn't hold it in. She stood me up, and we ran in place together.

"You are finishing something in these movements," she told me.

As I softened, the pain lessened. But with stress my body snapped back into its old shape. It took me years to notice, but the pain was in the same location on my body as my mother's pain. The same patch of flesh she bruised on impact.

A memory in the shape of my mother.

The opposite of a frozen body is one springing for flight. It's normal, she explained. Usually when a person comes out of freeze, they go into flight or fight. The deeper the freeze, the more aggressive the flight.

———

When I was talking to frozen women—women who experienced freezing or tonic immobility during a sexual assault—I started hearing stories about violent convulsions that started months or years later. Trembling, tics, drop attacks, seizures that were not epilepsy but looked exactly like it.

It started with Kim Corban, who told me she "froze in all the different ways one could freeze," and when we were talking she mentioned, as an aside, having convulsions—which seemed like the opposite of freezing. A year after the rape, she was having seizures that doctors told her were not epilepsy but connected to post-traumatic stress in the aftermath of her assault. "So I don't know if that's necessarily a type of immobility," she said, "but it was paralyzing. I didn't have control over my body."

The story began in the early morning hours of May 12, 2006, when Kim was a sophomore at the University of Northern Colorado. She told me how she woke up on her stomach with a shirt over her head and felt her own breath hot on her face. She tried to push herself up but was immediately pushed back down. A person was on top of her and she heard a low, taunting voice say, "Shut up. Shut the fuck up. Don't say anything." She felt a piece of hard metal touch the back of her head. "You need to stop being a little bitch," the man told her.

When had she been "a little bitch"? She couldn't think of anything.

On the wall hung a paddle from her sorority and a certificate from initiation. The night before, she had nailed framed photos on the wall of her boyfriend and her family—all the people who were important to her. On the bookcase there was a knife and a hammer and tools she'd used to hang up pictures. She had a goldfish in a bag.

He spent two hours in her bedroom, talking to her, touching her. There was nothing she could do. She tried to guess his body weight. She tried to catch a glimpse of his hands.

When he was done raping her, he sat on the edge of the bed and said, "Well, I feel really bad about this. This is just going to ruin my day." He said he was going to come back and do something nice for her. When he said it, he put his hand on her shoulder. Kim looked outside through a crack in her blinds at a blue hue, a predawn light. Then he leaned down and kissed the top of her head.

Campus police caught him three weeks later taking photos of his next victim. "But we learned later that he had tried to dance with us," Kim told me, "and we did the creeper shuffle away and pissed him off. He stalked us for a week and then chose when to break in."

The seizures started over Easter weekend in 2007, almost exactly a year after her rape, when she was preparing to go to trial. Kim was driving home from her boyfriend's house late at night, when she started feeling tense and strange, breathing quick breaths. She pulled over and called her mother for help, thinking it wasn't safe to drive.

Her mother, Deb Corban, lived in Loveland, just a couple

hops over and a straight shot down that road. She was on her way.

She drove all the way to the boyfriend's house but couldn't find her daughter. She looped back and finally spotted Kim's car on a side street. Deb helped Kim into the passenger seat, and by the time she walked around to the driver's seat, Kim was slumped over the console, unresponsive and shaking. Deb tried to get Kim conscious again but couldn't. She rushed to the hospital, and as soon as the nurses saw her, they put her on a gurney and tore off her shirt. Kim said, "Please don't!" And the convulsions became more intense.

Deb never thought to tell the nurses that Kim was a sexual-assault survivor. "It didn't occur to me," she said, "everything happened so fast."

That was the first of many episodes that weekend. Kim never saw them coming. She'd be sitting there talking and down she'd go. "It was horrible," Deb told me.

Deb dealt with it alone because her husband was away at work, driving a truck through a snowstorm in Iowa. Kim was having three to ten seizures a day. They lasted from a few minutes to hours. One of the longest episodes lasted three and a half hours. Kim didn't talk during the seizures. She kept hitting her head.

When Deb's husband returned home, he put Kim in a recliner surrounded by pillows to kneel on and they took turns watching over her.

Early on, in the middle of a convulsive attack, she sometimes relived the night of the rape by clawing at her face, thinking the shirt that the rapist put over her head was still there.

"I would wake up with bloody scratch marks all over my face," she said.

"It's like Kim would go unconscious and fight the rapist," Deb told me. "I would see her look at something in the room, a look like *Oh no, he's here,* and then she'd try to get away from it." The reenactments happened again and again.

After an episode, Kim often woke to bright lights, an aching head, lost memories. It took a while to come back—she could hear words but not understand their distorted warble. Occasionally she had to change her underwear, soaked in urine. Sometimes her head hurt because she was concussed, and other times because her muscles tensed too long.

The seizures started on Good Friday, and by the third day, Easter Sunday, she was admitted to inpatient psychiatric care and held against her will. They restrained her and double dosed her with Ativan. Deb remembered finding Kim in the fetal position with her arms around her knees while a doctor drew circles on a paper, saying, "This can happen, and that can happen," and Deb wasn't listening, and Kim wasn't listening, and a nurse said, "Did any of you guys want cookies or something?"

Deb was trying to explain to the doctor that her daughter didn't ever sleep alone and always needed the door shut and locked. So Deb was going to stay overnight. When the doctor told her she had to leave, Deb tried to check herself into the psych ward. She told them, "You can admit me too! I'm here to admit myself!" They ignored Deb, who tried to hang on to her daughter even as the doctors wrenched them apart. The women were crying and screaming. A nurse pushed Deb into the elevator as she reached for Kim. The memory later appeared in her dreams. Over and over, she's was swallowed by that blue psych-ward elevator as her daughter's face vanished behind closed doors.

That night, Kim slipped out of bed and wandered the ward

in her pajamas, searching for a phone. In the hallway she encountered a lady wearing a cat sweater. The lady was cruel. We don't have phones on until morning, the cat sweater lady said. Kim returned to her room and pushed a desk against the door. The door handles rattled. People were knocking, trying to get in.

In the morning, she had no idea where she was. The doctor said they had made a mistake—she could go home. Out the window of her room she saw the church where she would normally have been heading that morning to celebrate the resurrection of Christ.

"And once I was released," Kim told me, "I started having seizures again and was back at the hospital."

Kim's mother quit her job and her father took family leave. They bought a new mattress—king-size—so that Kim could sleep between them. ("That was the second mattress," Deb told me. "Kim's friends also bought her a new mattress right after the rape.")

The hospital bills added up. Kim couldn't be left alone, and she couldn't finish her classes. She had seizures in malls, restaurants, the yard, all over the house. Once, she had a seizure in a locked car and a stranger had to break the window with a golf club to pull her out. Deb recalled a seizure that happened when they were all together, talking and joking around. "And I just remember we were laughing about something and it felt good to be laughing. And Kim had to pee, but she didn't make it to the bathroom. Down she went, right there in the doorway, and started seizing. We were like, Oh my god! Oh my god!"

Ever since the psych ward, not only would Kim see her rapist when she had seizures, she also saw the lady with the cat sweater.

.   .   .

A diagnosis of epilepsy can only be given by a neurologist, and at Kim's appointment Deb remembered seeing a look like *Please help me* on Kim's face before a seizure began. A seizure in the neurologist's office almost always meant the patient didn't have epilepsy. A video EEG confirmed this—the doctors found nothing abnormal about her brain activity.

Then what was this? The doctor diagnosed Kim as suffering from something known as psychogenic nonepileptic seizures (PNES). The Corbans had never heard of it. The doctor explained that Kim's body was shutting down in response to stimuli that reminded her of the rape. She was too stressed, too overwhelmed to deal with the world. Things that normally wouldn't push someone over the edge were causing Kim to have seizures, including triggers like the blue light of morning.

Aaron Fobian, a professor at the University of Alabama at Birmingham, told me these seizures are "one of the most common diagnoses in outpatient neurology clinics, right behind headaches." Fobian explained that some patients were so embarrassed by the condition that they decided to stop speaking to their doctors. Others were angry that a diagnosis took so long, especially after they built their whole identity around a diagnosis of epilepsy. On average, a correct diagnosis took seven to ten years. Kim was lucky hers took only a month.

"A nonepileptic seizure can look exactly like an epileptic one," Selim Benbadis at the University of Southern Florida told me. "But sometimes they will convulse with asymmetry. They convulse side to side, head shaking, asymmetrical slapping, flopping, bicycling, shivering, falling over."

These seizures, they're not a specific disorder, Benbadis explained. These are physical symptoms caused by emotional distress. They are a subgroup of what used to be called conversion disorder and what the *DSM* now calls somatic symptom disorder. Benbadis is a seizure specialist, so patients come to him when symptoms manifest as seizures. For those with abdominal pain or diarrhea, they go to the gastroenterologist. If they have chest pain, they go to the cardiologist. If they have back pain, dizziness, shortness of breath, or a cough, they go to other doctors. "This is not unique to us," he told me. "But if you type the word 'psychogenic' into PubMed, it comes up as seizures, and the reason for that is we can prove it. With EEG video monitoring, we can determine what's epileptic and what's psychogenic."

There's a subset of experts and patients who don't believe the seizures have anything to do with stress or traumatic experiences, and they describe the seizures as a "functional neurological disorder." They are still searching for, and hoping to find, a physical cause.

Lorna Myers is a neuropsychologist in New York who has studied and treated psychogenic seizures for over twenty-five years. She met her first patients as a medical student at New York University Medical Center. The doctor in charge called them pseudoseizures, which is what they used to be called, and they were sending the patients to psychologists, but the psychologists didn't know what to do, and so they sent the patients right back to the neurologists.

"They just kept going back and forth. It just sounded horrible. It sounded very much like the Freudian conversion disorder patients," she told me, "but for whatever reason, they were no longer being seen in psychotherapy offices, they were coming to epilepsy centers."

She took it upon herself to treat these patients, and when she did, almost all of them recounted violent histories or psychological trauma. They had been to war, lived through difficult medical surgeries, survived sexual trauma or tremendous chronic stress. They were treading water, she told me, juggling too much for too long.

"The tension builds and builds in these patients because they are detached from their emotions and from their bodies, and then it looks very much like an explosion. It looks like all of this tension coming out in frantic movements and thrashing." After the explosion, Myers's patients will often say it felt like a release, and sometimes they will sleep. One patient told Myers how she tried to fight off the seizures, but it was more painful to fight them than to let them happen.

Among her patients with histories of sexual abuse, the seizures often looked a lot like the sexual assaults: a thrusting pelvis, eyes tightly shut, crying and fighting during an episode.

"There was one patient who had tried to fight off the person who assaulted her but failed," she told me. "You could see her fighting during the seizure." The patient was devastated because the sexual assault was there for everyone to see.

With psychogenic seizures, trauma is the main risk factor, Myers told me, but there's resistance to accepting that psychological trauma is behind the symptoms. "My sense has always been we should not feel ashamed for having developed a psychological disorder that was not our doing. Even if it's genetic, it's not our doing. Why are people made to feel ashamed of having something psychological? I think we should be outspoken about this. We should say, yes, this is what I have and so what? I could have cancer, or whatever. Why do we feel that it has to be hidden or kept in the shadows?"

The arguments between those who thought trauma and chronic stress were underlying causes and those who preferred to define the symptoms as a functional neurological disorder (focusing on how the brain networks communicated) made me think of a 2022 sexual-assault case in Colorado. A young girl had been kidnapped and kept in a basement where she was beaten, used for sex, and, like a circus animal, given peanuts for food. It was an easy case to win, but they wanted to get the guy on as many felony counts as they possibly could. The prosecution argued that the child suffered serious bodily injury (a felony) on a theory that her physical brain had changed as a result of trauma (as evidenced by symptoms of post-traumatic stress). They brought in Steven Berkowitz, a forensic pediatric psychiatrist, to testify that trauma, especially chronic trauma, can literally change the brain of a child. They were able to argue that her symptoms were on par with broken bones. "And so that's another way we're trying to help victims of trauma," one of the prosecutors, Arynn Clark, told me, "by making it known how serious and debilitating the aftereffects of significant assaults can be."

For some, the seizures started as a "frozen feeling" in the face, or numbness in the limbs, perhaps an ache in the ears. Or it started as a small tremble that then jumped like wildfire from one limb to another. One woman let out an enormous scream before she dropped unconscious. Another stood up and walked while she convulsed as if trying to get away from something. The seizures didn't always look like epilepsy. They manifested in the form of trances, arm raising, eye shutting, paralysis, vocal tics, and body tics. Sometimes it felt like ants climbing on their skin, or television static in their ears.

The first seizure might be a fluke, but by the second seizure doctors will start medicating for epilepsy. If someone's still having breakthrough seizures, they might raise the dose or add new medications. If a seizure doesn't stop, they're going to be more aggressive, because an epileptic seizure that goes on too long can be deadly. These medications don't do anything, but the patients have all the side effects. Sometimes they're put in an ICU and intubated, and patients have died.

Many women were told that they were faking the seizures. It happened to Samantha Woods, whose seizures started as "drop attacks" in the military. She was stationed in Okinawa but was struggling with anorexia, and when she was relocated to San Diego, she kept fainting and falling to the floor. Eventually, these turned into convulsions. She had been raped twice and reported "freezing" during the assaults. She told me she had memories of childhood abuse but could not articulate them. In September 2021, Samantha was sent to an inpatient military program for mood disorders. It lasted thirty days. She remembered being stuck in a locked concrete room with a door and a window and a tiny little bathroom. A camera looked down on her from the ceiling. She was here because she was having three or four seizures a day. But she was embarrassed to be having seizures in front of everyone else, so she stayed in her room. "They told me over and over again that I had control over my body," Samantha told me. "They told me to take my meds while I was actively seizing. I was crying. They really hurt me." During a really intense seizure she threw up while on her back, and it wasn't a little bit of throw up, it was a lot of throw up, and so she was choking, and thankfully someone was there to turn her on her side. In her Navy medical record, she told me, it still says that she has "fictitious disorder."

I talked to an eighteen-year-old whose seizures started three years earlier when they started dating a girl in secret. (Being a lesbian was taboo in their Cincinnati neighborhood, and they weren't out yet to their parents.) "It got very unhealthy," they told me, "and we would argue a lot. And it got to the point where it was sexually abusive. And I think that was the turning point. We didn't communicate the pain."

That's when the seizures started. But no one believed them, and no one validated their suffering. They finally got what they needed from a psychologist in Colorado named Afra Moenter, who told them the seizures were a "dysregulation between the brain and the body that leaves your nervous system all out of whack." They liked this way of thinking about the seizures and said it felt really good to know that they weren't faking them. "Because sometimes, when people say you're faking it over and over, you're like, Well, maybe I am?"

They started to get better, especially once they talked openly about their sexuality and their parents accepted them. "I think we want to be heard," they told me. "And I think the seizures are the body trying to be heard. And I just wanted to feel heard because all my life I've been told I'm sensitive or that I care too much.... The seizures were my body saying: I'm going to make you listen."

For these sufferers, history weighed on them, and made it even more difficult to be believed. They worried that people looked at them like they were possessed. Like they were daughters of the devil or dolls with sliding eyes. A hundred years earlier, they might have inspired a witch hunt.

A convulsing woman with an arched back—the quintessential image of Jean-Martin Charcot's hysterical women at the Salpêtrière Hospital in Paris—later became one of the most disturbing images of *The Exorcist*: when the possessed girl "spider-walks" down the stairs in her home, descending on her hands and feet, headfirst, stomach to the ceiling.

The ancient Greeks thought epilepsy was a disorder of supernatural origin—either demonic or divine. It was once called the "falling sickness" because a person in the throes of seizure would fall toward hell. *The Malleus Maleficarum*, the fifteenth-century treatise on witchcraft, called seizures a special characteristic of witches. Thirteen-year-old Martha Goodwin "was visited with strange fits, beyond those that attend an Epilepsy, or a Catalepsy, or those they call The Diseases of Astonishment." Locals believed she had been cursed by a witch.

Seizures have also been sexualized in ways that harm women. Hippocrates described "coitus" as a "slight epileptic attack." The sixteenth-century Dutch physician Johann Weyer described seizures as a form of pathological rage that was most likely to affect virgins and widows and could be cured with intercourse or marriage. One historian wrote, "The bodily behavior of a woman having a hysterical seizure" is remarkably similar to that of women involved in some group ecstatic or semi-orgiastic experience. He noted the disheveled hair, the tossed-back head, the rolling eyes, the arched body. Seizing women have been said to exhibit "lordosis," a mating posture of female mammals, when the lower spine is curved toward the belly, the hindquarters lifted.

A thirty-year-old artist living in Baltimore told me about the time she was on a family vacation when she sensed a seizure was coming. There would be a lot of twisting and turning, limbs jerking, or clapping. Sometimes her body would do a "worm move," or her legs would just start jerking, or her arm would swing up and she'd hit herself in the head. Her vocal tics were like animal alarm sounds, warning others of danger. She could hold the tics in like a sneeze, but at some point they were all coming out—she didn't want to scare anyone or cry with embarrassment. "So I get into my car and go have what looks like a fucking exorcism by myself in peace and quiet," she told me. "I made a lot of weird scary noises and it hurt my voice a bit. Then I felt better. I had to do all the movements and all the sounds just so I could go back into the world."

She thought the seizures and tics started after she was raped by a colleague. She remembered that when she met her husband, she couldn't have penetrative sex without throwing up. Slowly, over time, it got to the point where they would try to have sex, then they would stop, and they'd try again. Eventually, she didn't throw up.

"It's confusing—it used to be 'hysteria,' a disease that was for women. And now, the *DSM* makes it real, but on the other hand, there isn't enough research or information for it to be understandable. It feels like nobody gets it, including the people who have it."

———

After Kim Corban's rapist went to prison, she stopped having as many episodes. The last one was over a year ago. "Maybe because I finally felt safe," she said.

But Kim still feels like she hasn't found the perfect way to talk about it without people saying, "I don't get it," or "How are you having this much of a physical reaction over something that happened all these years ago?" And she tells them, "That's what my body does."

"There are more studies now about what our brains do to keep us alive," she told me, "and it sucks that this is what it is for me."

She does what she can to protect herself.

Kim always tries to sleep through that blue dawn light. "Such a beautiful thing gone wrong," she said.

· · ·

In 1862, the Salpêtrière Hospital in Paris became the epicenter of the study of hysteria, the mysterious illness then thought to affect half of all women. Psychogenic seizures were once thought to be a symptom of hysteria. Jean-Martin Charcot accused his hysterical female patients of imitating the seizures of epileptic patients at the Salpêtrière in order to get attention (he accused them of having dramatic, self-centered natures). He also claimed they were prone to making false allegations of sexual abuse. The patients commonly had extensive sexual-abuse histories. "In fact," the scholar Asti Hustvedt writes, "the so-called hysterical seizures were often abreactions of rapes."

Asti Hustvedt and Georges Didi-Huberman have described the sexual trauma perpetrated by Charcot and his doctors at the Salpêtrière. Charcot had his naked patients paraded in front of him by interns and routinely took nude photographs. He got them hooked on ether. At night, the interns regularly had sex with the women.

In 1875, a fourteen-year-old named Augustine was admitted to the Salpêtrière soon after being raped by her mother's lover. A doctor insisted her vaginal bleeding was simply her first menstrual period. The doctors at the Salpêtrière were familiar with Augustine, and already knew she was sexually abused by her brother and his friends, but they had blamed the violence on Augustine's loose morals (which they claimed were part of her hysteria). They monitored Augustine's vaginal temperature and secretions. Sometimes Charcot silenced Augustine with "an artificial contraction" of the girl's tongue.

Perhaps unable to speak directly about her rape, Augustine did so by other means. She reenacted her rape, had visions of "rapes, blood, more fires, terrors, and hatred of men."

Charcot made Augustine "gently sway her legs and pelvis"

as she aggressively recounted the details of her rapes and loves, showing the photographer everything: "That's how you make babies," she "confided" to him.

Augustine had a severe attack of hysterical epilepsy after being put on display at one of Charcot's teaching rounds when the man who raped her appeared in the audience. He went by the name of C. "This reaction was attributed to her psychopathology, and C was spared any blame."

Eventually, Augustine disguised herself as a man and fled.

When Charcot died in 1893, hysteria fell into the shadows, and so did public interest in women with convulsions. His team of doctors were laughed at. His disciples were exiled to distant wards, and the symptoms that were called hysteria became a thing nobody wanted to study. But we still don't know what to do with a shaking woman.

I have found a modern-day Augustine. Her name is Amanda, and she lives in Canada.

Amanda told me she started crying when I emailed her because no one had ever cared about what she was going through, let alone asked about it. She invited me into her home, at the end of a dead-end street on the edge of Lake Erie in the town of Kingsville, Canada's southernmost town. She lived in a small unit in a modular home with hardwood floors and inspirational quotes in every corner: "P.S. I love you," "We Can Do Hard Things," "Thankful for a house full of the loves of my life."

"I don't go many places," she said. "I go to safe places, I don't go to many new places." She missed putting on a nice outfit to go to work, brushing her hair, putting on makeup. She used to work as a teller at the local bank, and missed the older couples who chatted about their grandkids.

She wore yoga pants and a fleece. She had long blond hair and skin that hadn't known the sun. We sat across from each other on overstuffed couches. The ceiling was low and the lights were off. Behind her, across the room, small windows filtered winter light. On a table beneath the window was a large framed photograph of her eight-year-old son. She shared the house with her boyfriend, Drake, who was out taking their puppy for a walk.

"I just miss being out in society and making my own money," she said. She couldn't afford the gym anymore, so she took walks. She wanted to get back into yoga, but even then, sometimes she wondered: Am I feeling lightheaded because I'm doing downward dog or because I'm about to have a seizure?

She was not really fully with me in the living room. I could see it in her eyes. She was like a balloon about to slip free of a child's fingers.

She folded socked feet beneath her legs and sank deeper into the couch.

It all began in 2006, when she got a text message from her ex-boyfriend asking, Who is my son's father?

Amanda didn't understand the question, not at first, because her ex *was* her son's father. There was only one other person it could be, someone she had wanted to forget. Amanda checked her email: Her ex had sent her the DNA paternity test. He told her he swabbed the boy, who at the time was four years old, and sent the test off without telling her. The boy, he had decided, didn't look anything like him.

The news stilled her. After a moment, she rose slowly, methodically, and gathered some things—a bottle of lorazepam (a sedative), a pair of scissors, and her car keys. She got in her Jeep, the white one with a BABY ON BOARD sticker, and started driving. Soon she was on the back roads of Essex County, looking for a tree or a barn or a pole to crash into and die. She found a good tree but couldn't get a clear shot because there was a ditch in the way. She kept driving, chewing the lorazepam. At some point she took out the scissors and started chopping off all her hair—she had long blond extensions, a gift from a recent boyfriend. They were thick and tricky to cut. She had to really squeeze. When the police came, Amanda didn't look up at them. A lady officer was talking, but her words made no sense. Amanda stared at the hair in her lap.

At the psych ward, Amanda paced the halls in sticky socks and wondered, Am I going to look at my son and see the rapist? She had wanted to forget about the rape, but now it was like the rapist was coming back into her life. Should she tell her son?

"What do I do with this information?!" Amanda yelled. The words echoed. "Please help me," she pleaded. "What do I tell my son?!" No one answered.

Back at home, Amanda sat down with her son in the living room and worked on a coloring book. He picked a page with a mother giraffe and her baby. She cried because she regretted trying to kill herself. I'm here for him, she thought, I don't want to leave him, and how could I have done this to him? All she felt now was love. Knowing the truth about his biological father didn't make her love her son any less. If anything, it made her love him more. He was five years old. He was about to start kindergarten.

I asked how she told her son the news about his father.

"I just said something along the lines of, 'He's not your father and your real dad is someone who isn't going to be in our lives, and it's to protect you. And I understand if you're angry.' And he just looked at me and said, 'Why did you lie to me?' He was very angry. He said it a couple of times: 'Why did you lie to me? Why didn't you tell me?!' I kept saying, 'I didn't know. I didn't know, buddy. I would never have lied to you about this.' And he said, 'Who's my dad?' And I said, 'Buddy, he's not going to be someone who's going to be in our life. He's not a good person, and I'm doing this to protect you.'"

Sometimes she stopped responding. She sat motionless, her gaze locked on something in the corner of the room. We were silent, but silence was part of the fabric of her storytelling. Her jaw clenched ever so subtly. Her arms raised, and then again she started talking.

She was still working on changing the birth certificate. Her son needed a new legal name. It was a mess.

A couple months after the paternity test, she started having seizures every day, multiple times a day. They were the violent kind that looked like grand mals: fluttering eyes, groaning, violent convulsions.

Once, when she had a seizure in the shower, her body folded but her head was upright, and the water poured into her mouth. "Like I was being waterboarded," she said.

A doctor told Amanda she was only having them because people were around and she wanted attention. He said that if she lived alone, she wouldn't have them.

She felt trapped in her own body. "I have so much pent-up anxiety and trauma, and it's like shaking is the only way my body knows how to release it." The body in the act of escape.

Fighting when it hadn't fought. She had been raped by a man she met on a dating app and she had gone to his home, eaten dinner, and then he had pinned her on the couch. She froze.

Lately, she hasn't felt them coming on—she'll just drop to the floor unexpectedly. She never knows if she is going to smack her head, break a bone, fall off a chair.

"It's also hard to understand," she told me, "how something so great came out of something so horrific," meaning her son. "I had to go through something so horrible to get the greatest blessing of my life, and I wouldn't go back and change it because then I wouldn't have him."

When Amanda's boyfriend, Drake, came home, he joined us on the couch. Drake is a social worker and stand-up paddleboard instructor with dark hair and a beard.

They met on Bumble in June 2023, when Amanda didn't have much hope that she would ever meet someone (men stopped talking to her once they learned about the seizures). Drake was different—he asked a lot of questions and remained curious rather than dismissive. The seizures meant she couldn't really go out, so they had all their first dates at her place. After her son was in bed, they'd hang out in the living room and try to be quiet as they got to know each other. They took their time.

On their second date, Amanda told him her whole story. She told him about the seizures and the rape and the ex-boyfriend, and Drake did the same. He told her about his depression and drug use and how he was living without purpose after a divorce. But after a dark period, he went to treatment and stopped using drugs.

"I came into this relationship feeling like, here's my chance to show her that men can be good. It's my job to turn that story around for her, to change that narrative."

They were both scared of the other leaving. It took a while to learn how to care for each other, and for Amanda to understand that she wasn't a burden. Drake didn't see a seizure until they had been dating for three or four months, and he had enough love for her by then that it didn't change anything.

"Usually, I'm sitting here on the couch when I hear a thud," he said. He has to muscle his way around her convulsions to move her to a safe place. He was always putting pillows under her head. When they first started dating, she was having three or four seizures a day.

But one day she had six seizures, and Drake worried she was going to get brain damage, so he brought her to the emergency room. "I also learned not to bother ever doing that again; it's pointless. They just want to put her on medication. And the one doctor we had in particular was kind of demeaning."

They were deeply in love, and things had been going so well with Drake that one day Amanda decided to stop taking her antidepressants. Then she started having these dreams in which she wandered the house and swallowed every pill she could find; even during the day, she was still inside the dream, which was speaking to her and guiding her.

I was shocked when she told me: About two weeks before I arrived, she had decided that night was going to be the night she ended her life. And she did just as the dream told her to do: She swallowed every pill she could find—bottles of lorazepam and diazepam and even the extra antidepressants. She didn't want to wake up in the morning because she didn't want to keep having these seizures. Drake found her overdosed on the floor and brought her to the hospital. She ended up in the psych ward once again.

We were all quiet for a moment. I realized I was lucky to be talking to Amanda because she could easily have been dead.

"It's painful to watch her be in pain," Drake told me. "Every time I see her having a night terror, or being really bummed out after those dreams—it's hard to see her suffer because I know why she suffers. It makes me sad and makes me want to punish the people who did that to her. It just doesn't seem fair. Why her? What's the purpose of this? What's she supposed to do with this? How is she supposed to move forward and be productive in life? Even at night, she'll move around. She'll shake. I feel her moving her arms around and saying things like, 'Stop it,' or 'Don't do that to me!'"

Drake put the puppy down and crossed his legs. "It's disturbing," he said. "That's the word I'm looking for." He took a moment and then said, "What pisses me off is that this guy just walked away from this thing. Has he ever thought about it again? I can't believe someone else still holds this power over her. I just hate that. That's what I don't like knowing about her—as if she's not in control of her own emotions. It's like something else has the power over her, has power to come into our lives, our home, and infiltrate her day. Maybe he went home and told his friends and laughed about it. You kind of want justice or something, but I don't know even what could be done at this point. Would that bring the rapist right back to her son?"

"That's scary," Amanda said.

"Yeah, scary to open that box," Drake said. He scratched his beard and looked at his feet. "It really does freak me out a little bit when I think about her son. When he's eighteen, what are we going to do? I feel like it's his God-given right to know the truth. So I just feel like we got ten years to prepare for that."

———

Is there a value in trembling?

We know that women, after giving birth, tremble to relieve stress.

We know there are plants we eat to induce convulsions, and electric currents to produce shaking for the depressed and the schizophrenic and those suffering epileptic seizures.

We know that in 1237, hundreds of German children danced along the road to the town of Arnstadt. Their bodies were out of control, sometimes twitching or convulsing. In 1374, in the town of Aachen, hundreds of Germans began to writhe and whirl uncontrollably with a craving for dance. They danced deliriously until they collapsed and then complained of being oppressed until they were bound tightly in cloth to help them recover—and they didn't complain until their next attack, when they were hit with convulsions, panting, and foaming at the mouth.

The ancient Greek "Dionysiac cure" of dancing was not a series of simple movements of the legs, arms, and body, but a way to transport the self into another state of being—a way to cure phobias or anxieties.

We know that in the Taita Hills, where Europeans were rarely seen, the sound of motorcars, a train whistle, or the smell of a cigarette set off these seizures in local Kamba women. They said that the spirits responsible for the attacks came from Europe. Sometimes it was fear of the Europeans, but sometimes convulsions started because the women desired something from the men.

"A woman went into saka," wrote anthropologist Grace

Harris, "because her husband, having no cash, would not buy her sugar." She called saka "an illness of wanting." Men controlled their supplies, and shaking was a way for women to ask for what they wanted.

In an old *National Geographic* video, a polar bear is shown running from a helicopter carrying biologists who want to capture and tranquilize him. The bear, usually the apex predator, collapses into a state of tonic immobility. To come out of the freeze, his body trembles, his legs thrash, and his mouth bites the air. He looks like he's having a seizure.

The psychologist Stephen Porges was the first to recognize that wild animals sometimes tremble to recover from stress and that humans often suppress this natural process. We're told not to cry and to act tough. We're sensitive to the judgment of our peers. We try to process things later.

In 2008, a psychotherapist named Peter Levine met a Marine who'd nearly been blown up twice by IEDs in Iraq. Ever since the explosions, the Marine had been overwhelmed by convulsions that seized his neck, jaw, and shoulders. Often the man's hands automatically lifted to cover his face.

"The movements you are making," Levine told him, "are the kind of movements your body would have made if there were an explosion." Levine noticed the man's jaw clenched before the neck and face and shoulders. Levine had him open and close his mouth slowly. It was a small, intentional movement instead of an out-of-control movement. After a moment, the Marine felt a tingling warmth in his jaw. A sign of relaxation, said Levine.

"Almost like you got jolted out of your body," Levine said, "and what we are doing is calling you back into your body."

.   .   .

One summer I joined a class meant to teach students the art of trembling. The instructor called it "an experiment in giving up control."

A Catholic social worker named David Berceli came up with the idea that shaking might be a way to release trauma when he was huddled in a building in Lebanon that was being shelled by mortars. He looked around, and saw that everyone had assumed the same position: shoulders and hips contracted toward each other. Fear squeezes us into our smallest shape. Later, in another war, he was shelled again, and he noticed the children trembled but not the adults. Two days later, when he was alone and no one was looking, he began to shake. Had he tensed himself against his natural instinct to tremble? Have we been socialized out of trembling?

The instructor tells us it's the psoas muscle that contracts to bring the shoulders to the hips when we are afraid. It's about as wide as a fist and as long as a flute. If you eat a tenderloin steak, or filet mignon, you're eating the stress muscle of a cow That's what we are trying to release with trembling.

First, we tire our muscles with little exercises, and when it's time to shake, we all lie on our backs with our knees bent. The instructor tells us to lift our hips, and in this position we wait for the trembling to begin. "Eventually, the movement will come," the instructor says, "and when it does, you surrender."

There are about twelve of us, all women, hips raised to the ceiling, waiting to tremble.

I'm surprised the shaking comes easily, and it feels pleasurable even, like small, endless, nonsexual orgasms. I try to allow the tremors to be as big as they need to be. I try to surrender. Is this a kind of wildness? This freedom to tremble? Animals tremble in the wild and the instructor tells us that the trembling brings us closer to our animal selves. I think of myself in the forest again, rising from the ferns.

The wild is, as the poet Gary Snyder describes it, "elegantly self-disciplined, self-regulating. That's what wilderness is."

When Amanda posted a video on Instagram of herself having a seizure, Drake told me he was "flabbergasted." Amanda admitted the post was uncomfortable and surreal. It wasn't pretty, she said, but it was a way of controlling her image, which mattered because the images of hysterical patients at the Salpêtrière were often scantily clad women performing illness for an audience of male doctors. By posting the seizure, Amanda was taking control of what a traumatized woman looked like, which has always been controlled (and eroticized) by men. It was her image to capture and share.

A year later, Amanda wrote to tell me: "I'm better." The seizures disappeared—almost. She was just over two months seizure-free. It wasn't all good days, but it was as if some vital force had returned to her. We spoke over a video call and her face was caught in a sunbeam. She looked different. She was animated, already more alive. "I don't know if I told you this," she said, "but when I woke up in the hospital, I was upset that it didn't work. I was drained of hope. There was nothing left. And now I want to live and I have so much hope."

Her recovery involved therapy, new medications, a higher dose of antidepressants, a prayer group. "And I think our meeting was the beginning of exactly what I needed," she told me, "just that validation of someone caring outside of my immediate family and friends, someone wanting to hear my story and believing me. And now I know I'm not this horrible person, and I'm not defined by what happened to me, and I deserve a good life. And I'm going to do everything that I can in my power to make that happen."

Now, instead of convulsions, she experiences sleep paralysis, a semiconscious state that prevents the body from acting out dreams in REM. One can't move or scream, but often feels the threat of someone or something in the room. "I can't open my eyes," Amanda explained to me. "Can't talk. Can't move any body parts. But I have this feeling that someone's in the room. I feel like someone's about to grab my neck. I feel someone's hand on my neck, but I can't do anything."

I learn the rapist had choked her.

She was still trying to get rid of him.

But Drake is always there, next to her in bed. And that's what mattered in the end: Drake with gentle hands ready to catch her. She is slippery as a fish when she breaks free of the paralysis, wildly thrashing out of her sheets. All the movements she couldn't make, and didn't make when she was in the man's grip, like a squirrel in the talons of a hawk. The other man would go away one day. The day is coming, and he is almost gone.

Persephone, or To Bring Destruction

MEGAN SCHNETZER IS A SPECIAL EDUCATION TEACHER IN Delaware. She was raised a Christian and believed every-one should stay a virgin until marriage. She preached the sacredness of sex. "Sex was love," she said.

"But after the rape," Megan told me, "I went totally the other way. I just wanted to be fucked, you know what I mean? I wanted to be thrown around. I wanted to be choked. I wanted to be treated the way I felt. And my sexual preferences in the bedroom changed because of how I was assaulted. I remember one time my husband set up candles and had this whole thing and I freaked. I had a total breakdown."

Megan's husband sat her down and asked her to share every detail about the assault, but she didn't want to talk about it. She just wanted to forget and pretend to be somebody else.

"I couldn't stand living in my own body," she told me.

The man who did it had been her friend for fifteen years. She had grown up with him. They went to the same church. He was at her grandparents' funerals and she went to the funeral of his sister. She trusted him more than anyone.

Then, one day, he gave her a ride home and brought her to his apartment. It was the third or fourth story of a complex, and she didn't have a car. It was about 10:00 a.m. She was twenty-seven and married with a kid. He was also married with a young daughter.

She was held against her will in his apartment and was assaulted over the course of six hours. It was premeditated. It was slow with a lot of mind games. It started out with his approaching about sex and her saying, "I don't want that," until she realized it didn't matter how many times she said no. He didn't care. She was naked, and he would throw her clothes to the other side of the room and tell her that if she wanted them back, she needed to go get them. It meant walking across the room naked in front of him. He filmed videos of her doing these things to humiliate her. When he pinned her down with his hands, she found herself paralyzed and mute—in a state of tonic immobility.

Megan's friends and family pushed her to share all the details with a professional—and so she did what they asked and she met with a therapist and she told her story over and over again for two and a half years, and nothing changed. Mostly, after she talked to the therapist, she felt worse. After each session she went to a bar to drink herself into oblivion.

She would do anything to feel again—feel love, feel her body. Her two-year-old daughter meant everything to her, but now she didn't care much about what her daughter was doing. Megan was drinking too much and then driving. She was drinking too much and then having sex with strangers. She was watching porn and she'd never watched porn. It felt like someone else was taking over her body and doing these things without her.

"Sex was a form of self-punishment," she told me. "It was almost like, well, this sex is what I deserve, you know what I mean? A lot of victims feel unworthy, and dirty, and unlovable, and like they are pieces of trash, and honestly, that's how I felt.

I didn't feel like I deserved anything good. I thought I deserved to be treated like a piece of trash."

When people explained to me why they had sex again with the same person who assaulted them, or had sex soon after being assaulted, they often said it was because "this time it was my choice," or "I initiated it," or "I was going to have sex when I wanted with whomever I wanted." They explained how "it made the first time feel less like rape," or "it helped the first event lose meaning." They decided "it was a retroactive way of giving consent," and that the sex they didn't want and did not enjoy was "the only power" they had. They wanted to say, "I'm going to decide who has sex with me," and "I'm going to decide who gets to touch me."

"I had a case," prosecutor Arynn Clark told me, "where the victim was sexually assaulted, and within three days of her sexual assault the victim told me, 'I called up my best friend and I asked him to have sex with me because I didn't want the only experience I had of sex to be rape.' "

In one study of college-age women, about 50 percent reported having sex again within a month after sexual assault. In fact, many reported having more sex after their assault than before it. Women who were date-raped had sex more often and with more partners than women who hadn't been raped. Yet, among women in the study with rape histories, self-reported rates of sexual dysfunction were as high as 80 percent. The study specifically asked about risky sex—defined as compulsive sex, unsafe sex, or sex with strangers. The most common reason given for having this kind of sex after rape was for a feeling of "self-affirmation."

I remember reading in Annie Ernaux's *A Girl's Story* about the author's damaging sexual encounter with a camp counselor known as H. In the aftermath, H humiliates her by pretending she doesn't exist, and other counselors call her names. Ernaux writes the book in the third person as a way of distancing herself from the troubling story. After the violation, she feels a need to be seen in a way that guides her toward sexual promiscuity—or what looks like it. "Since H," Ernaux writes, "she has needed to feel a man's body pressed against hers, feel his hands, an erect penis. The consolatory erection." She is filled with more desire than ever before. "She is proud to be the object of lust, and quantity seems to be her gauge of her seduction value."

The psychologist Aimee Stockenstroom told me she has spoken to lots of clients throughout her twenty-five-year career who struggled with "hypersexuality" as response to sexual trauma. She introduced me to one of her clients, a mother named Jewel. She had delicate curly hair and thick glasses.

Jewel lives in Bumpass, Virginia, but all of this happened in Roanoke.

The story started back when Jewel was nineteen, a virgin, living in a trap house with a lesbian couple and their three children. It was a two-bedroom apartment, and one night they had a party. She was getting a tattoo done on the kitchen table, and it was her birthday. She remembered kissing the guy giving her the tattoo, and she remembered being very unsure about what was happening. And then she remembered waking up at about four in the morning stripped of her clothes and feeling disgusted. She took a shower and then lay on the couch until everybody got up and went home, and then she went to work the next day.

"And that was my first sexual experience ever," she told me. After that she spent a year having sex with as many women as possible, because she wanted to be in control. Women were physically smaller, so she thought she could overpower them. In this way, she was safe with them. "I became very promiscuous," she said. "I guess 'promiscuous' would be a good word, but I'm not sure." She paused and thought about it, then decided "promiscuous" would do.

She had sex with people she knew she wasn't going to ever talk to again. She enjoyed having complete power over someone, and then three hours later someone else. When she approached the women, Jewel acted dominant and aggressive. Nothing else mattered but having sex with them. She regularly ditched family plans and abandoned friends.

"I would drive an hour and a half to some random person's house to meet up with them. I did a lot of crazy stuff during that time." It was almost like an addiction, repetitive, on her mind all the time, taking over her life night after night.

She was partying more than she should have been and remembered missing work, and how her brother scolded her for it. She remembered one woman's house, way out in the middle of nowhere. No neighbors, no stoplights. It was really late when Jewel arrived, and she just turned around and drove back home. "Had I been older and wiser," she told me. "I probably would've felt unsafe more often."

Jewel told me that the sex empowered her in the moment, but after sex she was overcome with thoughts of self-destruction. "I worried about that quite a bit—the fear of being judged, and the fear of being rejected. And I very much kept what I was doing secret for a while in life. I guess I almost hoped that during that time somebody would've called me on it and been like, 'What's really going on?' "

. . .

145

In "Persephone the Wanderer," the poet Louise Glück writes, "Persephone is having sex in hell. / Unlike the rest of us, she doesn't know / what winter is, only that / she causes it."

According to Greek mythology, before Persephone was abducted by Hades, she went by the name Kore, which meant "maiden." She became Persephone only after the abduction—and Persephone means "to bring destruction."

———

In 2020, Saachi Gupta was living at her parents' house in Mumbai during the pandemic, and she didn't leave the house for over a year, not until her friend Nadiya had a birthday party in August 2021. Saachi didn't want to go because she didn't want to get COVID, but her friends told her to come anyway. If she didn't enjoy it, she could leave. She dreaded going and had a breakdown the day before the party. A month earlier, her friend Anika told Saachi that she had feelings for her, and it was confusing for Saachi, because she thought they were just friends.

At Nadiya's party, Saachi immediately got drunk, and so did Anika. Soon, they were all in the hallway, sitting in a corner together, talking and laughing. When Anika sat next to Saachi, she reached over and quietly squeezed one of Saachi's breasts, massaging it with her fingers.

"I thought, Holy shit, I have her hands on my tits and not in a good way," Saachi told me. And Anika whispered, Just say it if you want this. Saachi left and Anika spent the whole night crying and vomiting in the bathroom. Everyone had to take turns taking care of her.

Two days later, Anika texted Saachi, I was told that I behaved very badly with you, and I just think it would be good for us to take some space.

Saachi didn't want to give her space. They had been so close, and she wanted it to stay that way, but she also knew she should give Anika room to deal with whatever it was that had happened. Now, Saachi has panic attacks every time she comes across Anika's name.

Saachi wouldn't use the word "assault" because the word is too violent. She kept telling herself it wasn't sexual harassment; it was just that her boundaries were crossed. Her friends tried to tell her that if it was physical and she was uncomfortable, then it was sexual harassment. When Saachi came across an Instagram post about marital rape, it helped her think of what Anika had done to her as a violation—the same way someone you love and trust in marriage can still make you feel violated.

But there was no safe place to talk about sexual harassment except among the small group of friends and family she trusted. If her extended family knew about it, she wouldn't feel safe. The politicians in India were vocal about blaming victims for any kind of sexual harassment.

Three months later, Anika texted Saachi to let her know she was crying a lot and felt horrible about her behavior, and Saachi realized how much she missed Anika. She woke up for the first time in three months feeling happy again. She was singing in the shower, and she couldn't think about anything else.

But when Anika and Saachi spoke to each other over the phone on October 17 for three hours, Anika apologized through tears, explaining that she didn't think they could be friends after what had happened. The violation had changed the way Anika saw herself—she no longer saw herself as a good person. But Saachi thought they still had a chance to save their friendship, and she begged Anika not to block her. She hoped they could still talk or text sometimes. At midnight, they hung up. Right away, Nadiya called Saachi and asked her if she'd spoken to Anika. She said she had. How did Nadiya know?

"Anika accused you of making up the whole sexual harassment story and said that you had admitted that it hadn't really happened," Nadiya replied.

Saachi checked her text messages. Anika had blocked her.

After that, Saachi could no longer fall asleep in her bed, because it was where she used to text Anika all the time at night, and it reminded her too much of what she had lost. She had always felt the safest with Anika. It was different with other friends—if ever she'd had a falling out, she could look back and see the signs—but not with Anika.

Instead, she fell asleep in her sister's bed, but it was a broken sleep, and she woke up shaking. She skimped on hygiene, no longer brushing her teeth because she just wanted to fall asleep as quickly as possible. In the days that followed, Saachi couldn't stand being at home, and when she was, she would cry. She started drinking too much and ended up in the hospital. People thought that she should be getting better. And she was doing everything she could to get better. She was in therapy and taking antidepressants and antianxiety pills. Nothing was working because Anika was this person that she never thought she would lose, and now she was gone.

Eventually, Nadiya was cut off, in brutal fashion, by Anika as well, and she went from having a lot of friends to texting Saachi and saying, I don't have anyone to talk to.

A few months later, Nadiya and Saachi went clubbing, and when they got home, they started making out. Saachi had never kissed anyone before, but she wanted to get it out of her system. After that, Saachi started hooking up with random men. She walked right up to them and said, Do you want to hook up? Or she matched with them on Bumble and told them to meet her in two hours. She would hook up with anyone she could find. Sometimes she traveled for two hours just to see someone she had never met before. Mostly she went to their homes, alone. She knew it wasn't safe, but she did it anyway.

In the beginning, she wouldn't have sex with them. (She wasn't comfortable having sex yet because she was a virgin.) But they were often insistent and asked her repeatedly to have sex. Then, finally, she had sex, and after that she had sex all the time. She told her friends that she just didn't want to be seen as a person anymore—she just wanted to be an object.

"I was a fantasy," she told me, "like I wanted to become a fantasy for the men, and they could do anything they wanted to me, like tie me up, or fuck me in any way, and I thought I would get some pleasure from the act of sex, but then I was often incredibly bored, and I just looked at things in the room." She was mostly silent and didn't enjoy it, but she was also okay with all of it. There was never any attraction, nor any connection. There was nothing. A man tried to get inside her without a condom, even though she told him she wanted him to wear a condom, and he forced himself on her.

On the way home, she looked out the window of the cab and thought, Fuck, I did it again. Why was she setting herself up for more sexual trauma?

She went from being a virgin to having two years of consistently wild and unwanted sex, and she hated every moment of it. She made a list in her notebook, which she still keeps—a list of every man that she'd ever hooked up with. She had slept with thirty-seven people in seven or eight months.

"It's such a cycle," she said. "If something bad happens, you either hurt other people or you find ways to hurt yourself."

She spoke to a therapist about everything that she had done, and the way she had changed, and the therapist told her that "hypersexuality" is not just about having sex, it's about your entire life—your body language and behavior completely shift.

When we spoke, Saachi was still trying to be seen as someone other than the girl who had lots of sex for two years. The year before, for one of her classes, she made a comic strip focusing not on the act of sexual assault but what comes after it, and seeing it play out differently: how it is never perfect and never sweet.

Nadiya had a medical mask that she was wearing when she went to hook up with this guy who ended up sexually assaulting her, and she accidentally left the mask in Saachi's coat pocket. Saachi keeps it in her coat. She puts her hands in the pocket and feels the mask sometimes. The mask has so much significance for Nadiya, and it's such a heavy thing to carry around, and it feels good to carry it for her.

I Really Think I Love You

WHEN JENNA SORENSON TURNED TWENTY-TWO, SHE decided to move across the state of North Dakota to a town called Spearfish. She and her nine-year-old son moved in with her dad and his wife. Jenna got a job at a tattoo parlor. When she was drawing tattoos, she felt safe from the chattering anxiety that seemed to follow her wherever she went. She was hyperfocused on the drawing and nothing else. Then seeing people's faces light up after the tattoos—that was a beautiful thing.

After about a week in town, she got a friend request on Facebook from a local man. She accepted his request because he was good-looking, a bodybuilder, and she wanted to make friends. He sent her a message saying he was getting a tattoo from her boss next week and he would be sure to say hi. To Jenna, it seemed the bodybuilder had his life together—he was older, a business owner, and a parent of a little girl. He started bringing Jenna little gifts at work and he'd come see her every day at lunch. That's just what he did.

On their first day together, he said, "Check this out," and he showed her a taser and tased himself. Cool, she thought, so the taser doesn't work on him? It was weird, but she didn't know if this was a red flag.

She also didn't think the bodybuilder could hurt her because she'd already been hurt enough.

But any time she was free, he insisted on hanging out. She discovered an audiobook on his phone that was all about how to manipulate people, and he said it was for his business. He said he had two other houses in town, but she'd never seen them. He told her not to wear things with skin showing and not to post anything on social media about the two of them. He took videos of them when they had sex and sometimes she didn't even know it. She was miserable with him, but she got to meet his mom and his child and his sister, and that felt meaningful enough for her to overlook everything else.

When Jenna was in middle school, a lot of guys befriended her because of a rumor another student started about her being easy. Jenna was nice to the boys even after she realized they just wanted sex from her. "But," Jenna told me, "I just was hoping that one of the boys would actually love me."

When she got pregnant at fourteen, she didn't know who the father was because it could have been her boyfriend or it could have been the rapist. The rapist was nineteen, and he had been asking her for photos, asking her to come over. "Being groomed by older men was just a thing," she explained.

After having the baby, she went to get help at a mental hospital when she was only sixteen because she was nervous and deeply sad and she didn't want her problems to be her son's problems. I make friends with other people to get attention, she wrote in her journal at the hospital. I want to be wanted. I want to be valued. I change things about myself to please other people. After forty-five days of medication and therapy she got her mood up and they released her. She still ended up in a lot of abusive relationships after that. "So when it came to red flags and stuff, I didn't know. I guess at what point do I stop? At what point do I really know? Because it seemed to be that healthy relationships were just a fairy tale. They didn't exist."

One day in December 2020 the bodybuilder asked if he could sell the videos of them having sex. She said okay and didn't ask any questions because she didn't want to seem "crazy," which is what guys had called her in past relationships when she asked questions. She learned quickly to never push things. Questions meant anger and blame. She was the kind of person who really didn't speak up. And if she did, it was very brief and sort of quiet, and it really didn't seem to register with the bodybuilder because somehow the conversation would just wander in some other direction.

The first week they were dating, he wrapped his big hands around her neck and squeezed while he told her how hot she was and how much he liked her. You are beautiful, he said. She thought she was going to die. He said he wanted her to pass out, to lose consciousness, so that she could wake up next to his hard dick, because "that would be so hot." I'm going to die, she thought. She was sure of it. She hit his arms, but he wouldn't stop. That was her way of saying she couldn't breathe. She managed a little squeak, and he warned her not to lose eye contact with him. He wanted that eye contact. To survive, she pretended to pass out, which she assumed had worked because then he let go. But he turned to her and said he knew she was faking it. It was like she had done something wrong.

In the morning, she looked in the mirror and she seemed a bit purple, and there were blue dots all over her face, and one of her eyes was red, not veined red, but solid red, like someone took a paintbrush and swiped red paint over the white. Then the blood started seeping into the other eye. She decided that she had the face of a demon.

Even after all that, Jenna was certain there was something wrong with her because the bodybuilder said, "I strangle other women and they love it." She wondered if maybe he was just more experienced and that she still had a lot to learn. Maybe it was just something she had to get used to. It took a month for the blood to drain from her eyes.

When she no longer looked like a demon, she spoke up for herself. "You could've killed me," she said.

"That would've sucked for you," the bodybuilder said, "but it would have really sucked for me."

She tried to tell him that she didn't want to be with him. She tried saying how she didn't feel right with him, and that they didn't have much in common, and that it was okay that they didn't belong together. But he didn't seem to hear her when she spoke.

One night he asked her to come over and she said okay, so long as they didn't have sex. She wanted to sleep and lay down on the bed and try to relax. She had her eyes closed. He came over to the side of the bed. His dick was hard and he shoved it in her mouth. She was crying but said nothing else about it. When it was over, she told him that she was going to go outside for a smoke. She got in her car and left.

It was easier to express herself over text messages. The next day, she told him what he had done. He wrote back: Yeah, I was just being flirty.

Five days later, he asked her to come over again. He needed her ID to get paid for a sex video he'd shot of her. She was afraid that if she didn't go over he'd come after her for blocking his income. I'm just going to go over there and do this thing, she decided, and then I can be done with him. She stopped by in the morning, about five minutes before work so she had an excuse to leave quickly. He took a photo of her ID and then begged for sex. He took her to the bed and sat her down and undid her pants.

In the past, when he was drunk, he joked about raping her. And when he couldn't accept that she didn't want to be with him, he turned his jokes into reality. She didn't fight. He gave her a vibrator and she just took it and she used it. She wanted to get it over with and the vibrator would put an end to things faster than without one. "I just kind of let it happen, I guess," she said, not giving herself credit for the things she tried to do to keep herself safe.

"Looking back at this," she told me, "I just feel so stupid. I regret going over there, and I should have just listened to my instincts, but I don't know. I guess I was too naive to really understand what was going on."

When she first met him, she was off all her antidepressants and antianxiety meds, and had been for years, but now she has to get back on them and attend counseling again. If she misses one dose, she has a nightmare. In the nightmare, she's running from her rapist, although it's not really him. In fact, it's not really a specific person: It's all of the men she has known and thought she loved. In the dream she's running from them but feels trapped in the movement of the run. She wakes up in the night many times, but every time, when she falls back asleep, she goes right back into the dream. She could even be up for an hour or two before she goes back to sleep, and she'll still return to the same dream.

She is exhausted when she wakes up.

Before the trial, in the summer of 2022, she had been doodling and drawing at home and entered a trance state. She didn't know what she was making, it just came out: a woman, lying there dead because she got strangled.

Jenna was on the stand from eight thirty in the morning to four thirty in the afternoon. The bodybuilder still had videos that he made of them when they were having sex. The judge decided that it was okay for three of the videos to be played in front of the whole courtroom and in front of the jury. "Those videos had nothing to do with anything," she told me, "those were consensual." She admitted to using the vibrator, and the defense argued that it didn't make sense to use a vibrator and get raped. And so that was that.

"They were trying to say I was lying, and I was doing this for attention. Saying anything that they could to make me seem like I was some drugged-out, crazy, lying, attention whore. I'm being lied to about my own life. They went back and looked at what I wrote when I was sixteen at the mental hospital; how I didn't have any friends. It was so horrible. They told me I was claiming rape because I didn't like how I looked in a sex video. But I had never even seen it." Everything she had ever felt any shame about was on display. "The entire thing was absolutely traumatic. I understand now why people say they don't want to go forward."

The court decided that the bodybuilder was not guilty on the charges of strangulation and rape. Jenna came home and fell into a fog. Memories would come back to her in little spurts. She didn't want to be known for this. She wanted to be known for her art. "And so I've been really working on saying what I want to say when I want to say it and not being this scared kitten and just being more dominant, I guess."

Three months later she joined Brazilian jiujitsu, and it helped her feel more confident—helped her serotonin levels—but there were so many men, and when she tried to practice with men she couldn't do it because she couldn't think straight. She just kept imagining them as the bad guys, and she tried to calculate in her head how to escape.

Since the tattoo parlor is a few blocks away from the local gym where he works out, she knows he's often there, and sometimes she even sees him outside. There was one time when she saw him and their eyes locked.

One can see in Jenna's story the way love and loneliness can lead us to inescapable places, dangerous places. And that traumas can haunt future desires.

Mariana Bockarova is a psychologist at the University of Toronto who teaches a course on the psychology of relationships. A lot of the students opened up to her—either in class or later—to let her know they'd been in an abusive relationship or they'd been sexually assaulted and they were taking the class as a way to understand how to build a healthy relationship again. They all felt like they couldn't have, or didn't know how to have, healthy relationships with people anymore.

"In the aftermath of such traumas," Bockarova told me, "it's really difficult to go back to regulating as a normal person would. You have intrusive thoughts, avoidance, hyperarousal, hyperreactivity, and cognitive distortions—basically to make sure that you're safe and that you're in a safe space. If you've been hijacked by survival mode—your relationship is with the past more than the person in front of you."

When I met Mani, a New Yorker in his forties, he told me he had trouble forming relationships and keeping them. And yet, love was all he wanted. "I want a soulmate," he said.

We first spoke at a Sex and Love Addicts Anonymous (SLAA) meeting on a cold February night at the St. Francis of Assisi Church in Manhattan. The church is an old building with spires and crannies, looking like a candle that's been left out too long to burn and melt.

I found the "addicts" inside, sitting in a circle of chairs, in a room with nothing on the wall but a small painting of Jesus. The heaters hissed and clanked, let off steam, fogged up the windows. I could guess how tired everyone was by the way they held themselves. They rested their heads in folded arms or stared straight ahead with slack bodies. Some people were still wrapped up in scarves, coats, gloves, keeping themselves cocooned in fabric. Maybe they didn't want to be seen. It was a Friday, and the most dreaded holiday—Valentine's Day—was two days away. The city let us know how alone we all were, sending echoes of laughter up from the streets.

I was at this introductory meeting because I was curious to talk to the members. But I also wondered, Was I a love addict? What are they actually talking about when they say "love addict"? I'd always felt like love was the most important thing in the world, all-encompassing. I was a lover of romance. A lover of love. I was drawn to the stories of couples buried in the ashes of Pompeii, two people entwined forever. I had often found myself with men whom I didn't really know and who were not good matches and did not love me, and I found myself staying with them, waiting for love.

Pamphlets titled *Romantic Obsession, Withdrawal,* and *Healthy Relationships* were for sale in plastic bins. An introductory pamphlet warns that in the absence of this 12-step program people will be forced to choose between acute loneliness or addictive relationships, and this will set them up for suicide. I grabbed a quiz for newcomers, which was filled with statements to be agreed or disagreed with: Do you feel that you're not "really alive" unless you're with your romantic partner? Do you feel that life would have no meaning without a love relationship? Do you have a pattern of repeating bad relationships?

A recovered love addict wearing a beanie and sweatpants dragged a chair into the middle of the room. He was a former alcoholic but said love was harder to quit. Growing up, he had so many dreams; being a sex and love addict wasn't one of them. He took off his hat and put it back on. The addiction, he remembered, started on Valentine's Day in elementary school.

SLAA states on their website, "First you must face honestly that it is not simply 'the other person,' but primarily the neediness inside yourself that is the real source of the terrible pain."

Some people were still madly in love with someone who had rejected them, or someone who had abused them, or someone who hardly knew they existed at all. They were in physical and mental anguish. Letting go of a relationship felt like the world was coming to an end. They dropped out of school, embezzled money. They cut themselves, they overdosed, they abandoned family and friends. One ended up at the ER after an unanswered text. There were people who called their love interest a hundred times a day. Others dropped out of school, betrayed friendships, maxed out credit cards to pay for the relationship, or traveled to dangerous places.

The first meeting had me feeling lonelier than ever, and I tried to leave the moment it ended. But then a man walked up to me. It was Mani.

"Are you new?" he said and brushed his bangs away from his enormous eyes. He had pouty lips and a hairy chest that he let show above an unbuttoned shirt. His pants were tight and his shoes pointy.

"I'm in withdrawal," he said. He kept his eyes on the ground when he spoke. "I'm not really supposed to be talking to women. I'm not supposed to be making eye contact for more than three seconds with women that I find attractive, and well, I'm breaking that rule right now."

A few months later, Mani showed me the police report where he detailed the abuse he'd endured at the hands of a famous white man. He wrote about the day the man drove him home, parked in his parents' driveway, and held Mani's hand in a sensual way; and about the day the man lay naked with him in bed and touched his penis; and about the many nights he invited Mani to a local hotel and abused him. It started when Mani was a teen—the man was in his early forties. Unwanted sexual contact, including rape, went on for years, hundreds of times.

Mani suffered while the other man became successful and beloved. It's because of this abuse that Mani thinks he's never found love. He suffers from depression, feels shame. Why did this have to happen to him? Can he ever be loved? These are the questions he asks every day.

"Sex and Love Addicts Anonymous is not public enough," he told me. "People are so into their anonymity that they're preventing others from getting the help they need. These are intimacy disorders. The number one characteristic of a sex and love addict is getting involved with someone without knowing them."

On good days, Mani meditated, drank water, tidied his apartment, and listened to monk sermons. On bad days, he messaged fantasy women. His fantasies were the opposite of what he wanted in real life. In fact, he told me, "They are nightmares that turn me on." He had trouble getting work done because he just wanted to be in the fantasies all the time. "I'm talking to these women because I'm fantasizing about them," he explained. "I'm also talking to these women because they're far away. The women here, I might actually have to be their boyfriend. It's like I kind of want something more distant. It's a poor substitute for real love."

Sometimes he wrote down regrets in his notebook. Masturbation without love, he wrote. Orgasm without love. Premature sex. Sex before she's really your girlfriend.

SLAA gave Mani rules to live by. He wasn't allowed to look at women he found attractive for more than three seconds. He wasn't allowed to look at Facebook photos of a particular model he met on the subway. He was allowed to talk but not flirt with bank tellers, baristas, and store clerks. "They call it sobriety," he said, "but it's celibacy. It's emotional and physical anguish."

The withdrawal from fantasy can be bodily, full of aches and illness, followed by thoughts of rage, suicide, new addictions, and despair. It's usually when people fall apart.

"I had withdrawals from females much worse than any withdrawal from alcohol or drugs," one of the members told me.

"Grieve like they are dead," a sponsor recommended. "It is not a separation, it is a death."

Mani tried not to talk to women from nine to five on weekdays.

"Red-zone time," he called it.

When his therapist gave Mani the green light to date again, Mani showed him the profiles of the women he wanted to contact on OkCupid. They were all women doing headstands in leotards, whom the therapist called "narcissistic fantasy women who would never love him." Mani was impressed that his therapist could know this just by looking at the photos.

To show me how bad things were going, Mani played me a voice recording of one of his therapy sessions.

"They are rejecting you," the therapist said, "and that excites you. And that's perverse."

"I could fall in love with them," Mani said, "do all of this work, and then they could die."

"You are waiting for love," the therapist told him, "because you are afraid of it, and you are getting lonelier and sadder."

———

"You can tell my story," a love addict named Destiny said. "I kind of want to be famous, and we really need the publicity. No one even knows about us." Destiny is a twentysomething love addict with dark curly hair and big glasses whom I met at a meeting called "How to Become Unaddicted to a Person." She tried to leave her abusive boyfriend six times, but they always ended up back together. He insulted her, locked her up, slapped her. "On the one hand I was thinking, This is horrible," she said. "On the other hand I liked that this person was pining over me."

They dated for seven months—the longest she had ever been in a relationship. The whole time, he insulted Destiny, telling her things like how her hair smelled like Play-Doh or saying "Having sex with you on top is hard since I usually do this with small women." He always talked about his ex-girlfriends. If she tried to leave, he'd lock the door and stand in front of it. She couldn't say no to him. She would always see him even when she didn't want to see him. She cheated on him, hoping he'd leave her, but he didn't. The abuse escalated.

Destiny told me she had always had trouble understanding the difference between being sexually attracted to someone and loving them. And she would make herself think she was attracted to someone just because they were attracted to her. Then, as soon as a kiss would happen and "their teeth clinked," she would stop herself and think, What am I doing?! There were a lot of guys in college she tried to make her boyfriend. She loved the attention. But part of her was afraid of intimacy. None of the men she dated were emotionally or even physically available. She had lost her virginity to someone in a foreign country and was devastated when he broke up with her a month early, even though they were going to break up a month later anyway. "And then once I dated a man who was very weird. I had this fantasy that he was this brilliant writer and I was his muse. Well, that wasn't true. Fast-forward to being in New York and trying to find love. I'm just not hot enough."

When she finally thought she had the strength to leave her depressed and abusive boyfriend of seven months, it was almost like he sensed it, and he was at her apartment waiting for her. He said he wanted to break her nose, and then he slapped her. She ran away—out the door and onto the street. She caught a cab and told the driver to take her directly to an SLAA meeting. They told her that her case was extreme, and she should check herself into a trauma treatment facility in New York. She needed locked doors and security to stay away from the abusive man she loved. She stayed for ten days. That was the beginning of what she calls "no contact."

"If I didn't do anything," Destiny admitted, "this would be my entire life."

Meg is a comedian in Los Angeles, and for years all she did was cry, talk about men, and fail in her relationships. Men would tell her that they didn't want a serious relationship and she would stay with them anyway, holding out hope that they were the one, because they were *just so magical*. Meg told me about the time she was dumped but didn't accept the reality of it. Her first thought was: You are going to see me. She hung up the phone and ran into the middle of traffic on Sunset Boulevard to try to catch a taxi. She didn't want to waste time, so she stepped in front of a moving taxi, and it stopped just before it hit her. She was a little bruised and scratched up when the cab dropped her off outside the man's house. She was drunk and covered in blood, and he did not take her back.

When she wouldn't stop crying, a friend in Alcoholics Anonymous told her she might want to join Sex and Love Addicts Anonymous. Meg had never heard of it, and she wasn't excited about it. At the time, she was having an affair with a married man, dating multiple people on Tinder, and thinking she was in love with a guy friend. She weighed ninety-three pounds and was completely out of her mind attached to another person. She imagined everyone at the meeting was going to be a pervert, but she was desperate and went anyway.

The meeting was in a drab room in a church. Everyone said their name along with their affliction. There seemed to be so many afflictions: love addicts, sex addicts, romantic obsessives, intimacy addicts, fantasy addicts, emotional anorexics, intimacy anorexics. Meg didn't know what she wanted to call herself and so she said, "I'm Meg. I'm new." When the meeting was over, she left without talking to anyone. She wasn't taking it seriously—she kept drinking and dating men who treated her badly. She started hooking up with a guy she met in the comedy scene. He was a recovering sex addict, and one morning she woke up on his floor after falling unconscious from too much drinking, and that's when she decided to get serious about the program.

She preferred the women-only meetings. It was usually a group of fifteen to thirty people crammed into a room at a church. Meg noticed that most people at the meetings introduced themselves as sex and love addicts, but she didn't really relate to the sex part. A year passed before Meg introduced herself as both a sex and love addict.

"I still don't totally relate to the sex addiction," she told me. "But I confuse sex with love, and love with sex. So I'm a love addict who uses sex to get love."

She was paired with a sponsor, an experienced member who guided her through a recovery plan. And as part of this plan, Meg was told to avoid contact with men for ninety days, especially men who were ex-boyfriends, men she found attractive, and men she'd been involved with in the past. It also meant no conversations with any man for more than two minutes, and during those two minutes she wasn't supposed to reveal any personal information. Meg also stopped going on dates. As she made her way through the program, an acquaintance asked her out on a date. Meg liked him but had to tell him she was unavailable until she finished the 12-step program. If men reached out to her, she ignored them or explained to them that she was in a recovery program. They'd have to wait.

"It was brutal," she told me. "It was really painful. I was afraid men weren't going to like me anymore."

The acquaintance waited eighteen months. They started with one coffee date a week, and after a couple of months, two dates a week. She didn't let him come into her apartment until they were a couple. They didn't have sex until they decided they loved each other. The first time I spoke to Meg, they were moving in together. The second time I spoke to Meg, they were planning a wedding.

"Sadly," she told me, "it's part of our culture. You think you're supposed to be hooking up with people all the time. You hear: Just hook up with him! It's not a big deal! But for me, it ate my soul away. I didn't actually want to be doing that."

. . .

"You know romantic movies, romantic comedies?" Andrea Owen, a former love addict turned life coach, told me. "Well, that's our real life. We believe in falling madly in love on the first date and in love at first sight. If we have an amazing first date, then we become obsessed with that person. You know when you break up and you are sad because you are alone? Well, for a love addict it's about ten thousand times that."

She stayed with her ex through rumors of affairs and long nights where she didn't know his whereabouts. She wanted to leave him, but she couldn't do it. When she was thirty-one, he impregnated their neighbor.

After the divorce, she had a lot of trouble meeting men who cared for her. She dated a man who lied about having cancer to cover up an addiction to opioids. She dated abusive men over and over.

Abuse, neglect, or drama—it was all mistaken for intimacy.

I felt an affinity with this kind of longing.

I remember dating one person after another for many years without really knowing them, and then being devastated when things ended.

Friends had often asked, "Why do you keep dating these people who don't care about you?" But also, "Why do you date people you don't even seem to like?" Those people were proxies of companionship, salves for loneliness. I was a woman who could sustain a fantasy of goodness or compatibility or connection.

I stayed with a man who lived on another continent, and even though I rarely saw him, I spent thousands of dollars I did not have to fly across the Atlantic to see him, even after finding his backpack filled with condoms.

I stayed with the man who lied about being addicted to drugs and who vanished for weeks at a time and who snorted so much cocaine that blood leaked out of his nose like a fountain and splattered all over my face. He talked of ex-girlfriends and ex-ex-ex-ex-girlfriends and there seemed to be so many of them. The relationship was sustained by drugs and drinking and there were great voids of time spent together, talking about things I will never be able to remember.

I stayed with a man my friends said was always yelling at me, but I didn't remember him yelling. Maybe I disconnected from those moments.

I stayed with the man who announced to me that everything around him was always self-destructing. And when I was with him at the airport the parking ticket machine broke, and at home the sewage pipe broke and filled the basement with shit. He had been to war and was obsessed with war. I was so broke that I took out a $250 loan from the bank just to go skydiving with him, even though I don't like planes and I don't like skydiving. I just hoped the skydiving would bring us together.

The critic Helen Lynd once wrote, "The exposure to oneself is at the heart of shame." Exposure not only of oneself to another person but to a self that you hadn't yet recognized— or else ignored. We assume that we are one kind of person living in the world, until we discover we are something else altogether. Shame is when you stare at your past self, and she stares right back at you. That's how I felt hanging out with the love addicts.

The scholar Lauren Berlant has written that "to intimate is to communicate with the sparest of signs and gestures," but must also involve "an aspiration for a narrative about something shared, a story about both oneself and others that will turn out in a particular way." Sometimes we think people are connecting to us on a much deeper level than they actually are.

In past relationships, I'd always felt a bit like I was narrating the space between us, forgetting about myself, about my thoughts—that I even had them. Maybe because of the power some people inherit, they feel a need to engage, and so people like myself forgo our own comfort to comfort them. It's how many girls are raised, and how I was raised.

Berlant's intimacy describes a call-and-response—a way of being in a healthy relationship that I began to know only after I met my husband. It was such a simple thing. If I needed something, he gave it. If I was hurt, he attended to it. If he held my hand, I squeezed back. Our lives and bodies conversed and chattered. We shared a story, and until I met him, I had never had a story that was shared.

On a spring day in Midtown in 2018, I met Mani at a vegan restaurant. His beard was shaved, but a long, drooping mustache remained. He was dating again, he told me, "sober dating," under the supervision of his psychiatrist.

"Do you think you *actually* want to be in a relationship?" I asked.

"Yeah. I want a soulmate. I'm at the age now where I'm very sensitive. I have nineteen ex-girlfriends. I forget how many of those lasted a year, but that's the average length."

We were meeting his friend Scarlett, a woman he met at a party; they'd discovered right away they were both love addicts.

"We had vegan lunch yesterday, but she needed to go home to print something and needed my help and so I went home with her. She said she wanted to go to sleep, so I slept beside her and we kissed. We kissed on the cheek, but that was way too much for me," Mani said.

Scarlett told Mani they could be special friends, and that she could have one special friend at a time, but she couldn't have a boyfriend.

"I would sleep with her if I were her boyfriend," he told me. "We could do anything."

Scarlett arrived, a beautiful vegan with long blond hair and a wide mouth. She had just moved to New York from Florida and has been in SLAA for about a year. Mani sat with his back against the wall with his legs stretched out, one foot on top of the other. He looked at the floor.

"All I've ever wanted," Scarlett said, "is to be in a monogamous relationship, and all I've done is sabotage that. I sabotaged every opportunity that came to me because I didn't know what it looked like to be in a healthy relationship. I was the perfect person to walk into an SLAA meeting. I was sexually assaulted when I was five—like I had a dick in my mouth when I was five—and that's not easy to rationalize as a five-year-old. I was assaulted again and again until I was nineteen. I carry that."

Not long ago she had a boyfriend who told her she wasn't enough. He invited her over and refused to have sex with her and then kicked her out. And he didn't want to hold her hand in public. Lots of games, lots of abuse, until the relationship broke her, and in its wake, she stopped being able to have relationships at all. She said she would fuck people and leave them because she swore she'd never open herself up again to intimacy. She wouldn't let men see her in the morning hours after she fucked them.

"But the whole objectification thing I was doing to men wasn't really how I was feeling," she told me, "because I actually always felt a deep affection for them."

The waiter brought plates of steaming curry and rice. We ate in silence.

"I want a soulmate," Mani said again. "That's all I want."

"I want a soulmate too," Scarlett said. "It's the first thing I wonder about someone. I just look across the room and think: Are you my soulmate?"

"Remember," Mani said, "we were supposed to talk to the psychic? She's coming—she's ready to see us."

"A psychic?" I said. I imagined a woman in a long dress with bangles.

"Yeah, there's a psychic. She is going to see what our connection should be, right? We've got to see what the psychic says."

The psychic would tell them whether they had a romantic connection and if they should be together. They needed the psychic because they couldn't figure it out themselves.

"Maybe she should see what our energies are separate and then together," Scarlett said.

Mani straightened his back and squinted. They stared out the window together, by the doorway, the one that overlooked the sidewalk, bright with sun. Mani checked his watch.

"The psychic is running late," he said. "We need her." He looked over at Scarlett. "Don't worry. We'll know soon." They smiled at each other and Mani turned to me. "You'll have to go," he said. "It can only be me and Scarlett."

Outside, I glanced once more through the window at the two of them together, waiting to be saved by another story.

———

At the beginning of #MeToo, Jessie Ford, a sociologist at Columbia University, heard about the horrible statistics—that one in four college-age women would be assaulted by the time they graduated. The stats came from sexual-assault surveys, which asked people to check boxes. There was no room for narrative. So Ford wanted to know what people were really talking about when they checked those boxes. She did her own surveys with the same standard questions (asking about forced sex, incapacitated sex, pressured sex, pressured hand jobs, or fingering someone), but she also gave students a chance to tell their stories.

Ford's first interviews uncovered a range of sexual experiences described as unwanted, but none of them involved physical force, and only a minority involved the fear of such force. "What people were saying," Ford told me, "was so much more complex and layered than the stories we were hearing from #MeToo, and sometimes people literally didn't have the words to describe what was happening." She was fascinated, and spent almost another decade interviewing students, including straight men, gay, bisexual, and queer students, about "unwanted consensual sex," which is agreeing to sex one doesn't desire in the absence of coercion.

The more students she interviewed, the more patterns emerged. There were some stories that clearly depicted rape or assault, but the majority described having sex to fulfill social norms. They described ordinary concerns—feeling awkward or embarrassed—and how important it was for them to be "nice." They didn't want things to get "weird" or "awkward." Women worried they would be called a "tease" or a "bitch," so they gave hand jobs or blow jobs—anything to get out of the room. Even when there was no violence, the possibility of violence was always lurking, and sometimes this meant having sex they did not want.

One of the women interviewed for the study was Penelope, who was nineteen and a college sophomore: "I really don't know how to say no when a guy wants to have sex, I feel terrible when I say no. . . . Don't want them to see me as someone who doesn't want to have sex. At the same time, don't want them to see me as weak."

"They kept saying they felt forced by the situation and not the person," Ford told me. It meant feeling pressure to perform gendered roles. Ford was surprised. These were women who thought of themselves as equals in the classroom—in every aspect of life—but with sex, Ford told me, they lost that power, or the power changed. "They thought they were free of these gender norms, but the norms were very much in their heads."

The sex was "kinda terrible," Hannah, another student, admitted to Ford, but decided going along with it anyway made her "selfless," since the pleasure was "all for him." She was a bisexual college sophomore. It took an hour for the sex to end, and she was just waiting and hating it.

Cynthia, another student in the study, described how things went straight from kissing to vaginal. She didn't want to have sex, but it was too late. When he couldn't get hard, it was upsetting to her. She told him to take off the condom because she felt she needed to maximize his pleasure. They had unprotected sex. Later, she worried about pregnancy and texted him to ask if he came inside her. I think so, he said. Can you get me Plan B? she asked. Sorry, he told her, but he was out with his friends.

Jackie, an eighteen-year-old freshman in the study, had sex with a man simply because he was "looming." His physical size made her think about the possibility of violence, even though he was never violent and never forced her to do anything. But for her, at the time, it was better to have sex with him than risk any possibility of violence. "Consensualish," she called it. "Consensual but unwanted."

Men's stories weren't all so different. The men talked about having unwanted sex because they felt too awkward to stop things, or because it was "mean" to say something. They worried people would question their sexual orientation or laugh at them if they didn't have sex anytime it was offered to them. A college freshman named Mark, twenty-one, explained that one day he woke up to find a woman on top of him, trying to have sex with him, but he didn't want to make a big deal of it. Instead, men like Mark reported going through the motions and some faked orgasms to get out of the room. They also had the idea that men couldn't be raped, and it was confusing for them to imagine themselves as a victim, even when they were.

Many men's descriptions suggested that they were upset by the experiences but not sure how to express it. And so they used hypothetical role-reversal to express themselves— they often said if the same event had happened to a woman, they would consider it sexual assault.

College-age gay men in the study (who had rates of sexual assault and unwanted sex that mirrored the rates of straight women) often reported finding themselves without a script, and so they reverted to the only script they knew—pleasing the person with more power, giving orgasms without thoughts of their own. Lesbian and bisexual women had the most success escaping gendered scripts. "Queer women talked a lot about what they felt in their own body," Ford told me, "while straight women talked more about men's bodies or their own body as an object."

Ford wanted to know why "assault" was the only word available to describe unwanted sex when it was so much more textured and varied than that. "If someone knows an encounter didn't quite feel right then that's a good thing, but it's maybe less productive if the only way to describe that encounter is assault. Why not also talk about uncomfortable, consensualish, embarrassing, disgusting, painful, or creepy sex?"

And these encounters often felt deeply violating in their own particular way. Robin West, a professor of law and philosophy at Georgetown, named this harm "consensual sexual dysphoria"—when we violate our own sexual boundaries, sometimes betraying ourselves, but with reason and agency to accommodate another. And I found comfort in this idea of self-betrayal—it felt so true for many of my experiences, but hardly discussed. Sometimes we don't understand our own boundaries, much less articulate them. There can be a part of ourselves that is agential but also deeply lost and uncertain about what is normal.

Another Sleeping Beauty

Aaron hardly knew the woman, but he was certain Anne was the one he would love forever. Even after the relationship ended, which it did, Aaron never gave up his fantasy of being with Anne.

I met Aaron through a mutual acquaintance in 2017, and I was hoping to write a story about his experience in the military, but then he kept talking about Anne. Soon, all I wanted to do was talk about Anne too. We talked about Anne at night, over the phone, while Aaron was in Colorado and I was in Florida teaching at a writers' conference. He wanted to talk every day, or close to it, to get the story out as quickly as possible without long gaps between conversations. He didn't want it to drag on because the memories were painful.

I kept the windows open to cool the apartment and I heard animals moving around in the trees.

Aaron said they met as college students when he was twenty-one and she was twenty, at the Sun Bowl in El Paso: a weekend of college football, marching bands, and banquet dinners. He was a shaggy-haired wide receiver for the University of Missouri, and she was a sorority girl with long dark hair. When he saw her, it was as if he had traveled to El Paso just to meet her. They spent hours kissing in the car listening to My Chemical

Romance on repeat. They slept in the park or cheap hotels and blinked awake in one another's arms. They spent a few nights together, and then a few more. He took his scheduled flight home but returned to El Paso the next weekend to see her. He wrote her initials and the El Paso zip code on his arm at football games. He started to apply himself at school, considered a career in medicine, thought for the first time about leaving Missouri.

They didn't date for long, all long distance. With her in El Paso and him in St. Louis, communication tapered to a halt. They dated for six months and then it was over. He couldn't explain exactly how it ended, but it ended slowly, like a receding tide.

A decade later, he still loved her.

Aaron still had artifacts from their time together: a boarding pass from El Paso to St. Louis, a bracelet with beads bearing the faces of saints, a copy of Richard Linklater's *Before Sunrise* with a purple Post-it note that read "watch before sunrise." A card from Anne that read: "I've never been happier with anyone than I have been with you. We will find a way to make this work, I promise."

He couldn't shake the idea of her, not for a moment. He couldn't let her get away. The loss of Anne made him look at himself and think of himself as a schlub with barely passing grades. He didn't try to convince her to get back together right away because first he wanted to change himself. He agonized over what to do. One night he saw a headline about how a team of Navy SEALs killed Osama bin Laden, and he thought: If I were a SEAL, maybe I could get her back?

It took him two years just to prepare for tryouts. First he had to finish boot camp, technical training, battle stations program. And about three weeks into the twelve weeks of

Officer Training he started to feel sick. Eating a simple meal left him in agony, and he found blood in his stool. While you're in the military, you're only allowed to be seen by a military doctor, and if they find out that something is wrong, you risk a medical discharge. So he ignored his symptoms and ate as little as possible for nine weeks. After graduation, he went to see a civilian doctor who gave him a diagnosis of severe ulcerative colitis—an incurable autoimmune disorder. "The body not recognizing itself as itself," he explained. It was something he'd have to manage forever. He took steroids to suppress his immune system and saw a doctor in secret on the weekends.

The disease made his skin delicate, prone to bruising. His back bled after the first sit-up. Sometimes he defecated ten times a day, always with blood. Once on a run, his commanding officer walked up to him and said, "What the fuck is wrong with you?" Aaron was covered in blood, defecating on himself, bent over in the sand, and he had no response. It was freezing and the ocean was in a rage. He refused to admit that his body was breaking down, even while the commanders sprayed him with hose water and told him to roll in the sand, tread water, carry boats and logs. Aaron kept going. It was all for Anne, he thought. He paddled in the surf, tumbled in the white waves, and kept going until he blacked out on a rope climb and fell twenty feet. He hit the ground and started convulsing. When he woke up, he was on a stretcher with his neck in a brace. A rumor spread that he had died.

They rolled him back to the next class—which meant he would have to wait ten weeks for it to start. All he could think about was that it meant ten more weeks before he got to talk to Anne. Aaron convinced himself that Anne would love him if only he did this one thing. He had it in his head that Anne was waiting for him on the other end of Hell Week—the final and most difficult week, the week most everyone dropped out. If he made it, he believed, he would have the chance to talk to her again. Every step forward was one step closer. To keep himself going he recited lines from their love letters and sang the song that was their song. It helped him keep track of time, and helped him stay focused on Anne.

On his second try, he made it to Hell Week. From Sunday evening to Friday afternoon, they exercised twenty hours a day, ran two hundred miles, and barely slept—just four hours one night and thirty minutes another. The week began on urine-stained cots on the beach. He remembered one of the lieutenants saying: "There's a darkness inside you that you don't know about yet."

On Monday night, it all came to an end. They were jumping off a pier, over and over again, into the ocean. Aaron had two herniated discs and couldn't lift his head unless he used his hands to hold it. He couldn't keep his head above the water, but he imagined Anne was calling his name, waiting with open arms. He could no longer remember the words to their song. He prayed to God that his heart would explode—in the water and after, so he wouldn't have to quit. He was like a prince, tearing his way through the briars, covered in scratches, tangled in thorns. But he couldn't do it—his body was failing him.

When he got home, he pounded on the kitchen counter. "I don't know what I'm going to do," he cried as he wept on the shoulder of his roommate. "I'm not going to find Anne."

I interrupted his story. "Wait," I said. "You didn't tell her about any of this? She didn't know?"

"No," he said. "I didn't need to tell her because it was a story I'd tell her later."

Talking to Aaron was like talking to a character in a book.

There were conversations with phrases I felt I could only cite from a romance novel: "I would burn heaven and hell down if that meant I could be with Anne," or "I would set fucking heaven on fire in this life or the next. I will do whatever it takes," and "I promised her I'd change the world to prove how much I loved her," or "If my heart exploded it would be such a pleasurable way to die. I wouldn't have to feel anymore."

After Aaron was discharged from the Navy, he ran away to Montana, to desolate and beautiful places. He ran marathons, increased the miles, upped the difficulty of the terrain. He was a boxer in the ring, taking hits. He did five marathons in five weeks. In 2013, in July, he signed up for a fifty-mile ultra-marathon in the Mojave until it was canceled because of a heat wave. Aaron decided to run it anyway. Everyone thought he was chasing a challenge, but he just wanted to die. He had been thinking about ways to kill himself but didn't want to put his mother through it—he figured suicide by running would look like an accident. "I wanted my heart to explode," he said. He ran it when the sun was high and temperatures boiled to 117. On his chest he wrote: DO NOT RESUSCI-TATE. He was running to resuscitate Anne, to bring her back to life. If he couldn't do that, then he would die.

Somehow he survived.

A week later, he got a letter from the Marine Corps saying they'd accepted his request to enlist.

He smiled and jumped back into training. He was doing well, moving up the ranks, and was a few months away from a deployment to Iraq, when all the stress made his colitis flare. He vomited every morning and ran to the bathroom ten times a day. Often he cleaned his clothes of blood and mucus as much as he cleaned his rifle. He spent a weekend on his apartment floor, crawling between his bed (a camping mat) and the bathroom, barely able to breathe. His stomach was hard and distended. On Monday, he was in an ambulance, high on morphine. He remembered a spinal tap, CAT scans, MRIs, a colonoscopy. The official diagnosis took a couple of days—it was Burkitt's non-Hodgkin's lymphoma, stage 4. On the MRI, the cancer was everywhere, his lungs, his groin, every organ freckled with tiny tumors, all lit up like a Christmas tree. When his mother arrived, the doctors said they were going to take him to the brink of death and slowly walk him back.

Aaron looked at himself in the mirror. There were all these devices hooked up to his brain, including a chemo port. They needed to put the chemo in his brain, but since there was fluid around the skull, they had to take some out before they put more in. But they couldn't get the fluid out for whatever reason, and it felt like they had to force the chemo in. He lost seventy pounds, his hair fell out, he stopped looking in the mirror. There was a drain on his back and a catheter on his liver. He was helpless, days at a time, defecating on himself. Lots of OxyContin. He couldn't sit up, and if he tried to walk, he fell over and woke up on the floor. Sometimes he dreamed that he was running through a burning labyrinth, and when he woke up screaming, he licked the taste of sulfur from his lips. Every night, he had the same dream.

He showed me photographs he took of himself in the cancer ward when he was his loneliest self, trying to keep track of his disintegrating body. A photo from the morning he was diagnosed: giving a thumbs-up to the camera with a buzz cut. There are seven IVs above him, all lined up on the crucifix of a metal pole.

He took a Polaroid of his face—pale and hairless, like a gentle and beautiful bird. On the bottom he wrote: I'm still here.

"Even if the hair never grew back, even if the weight never returned, I wanted Anne to remember the person behind the alien in front of her," he explained.

He thought of putting a gun in his mouth and hearing the bullet break through his skull, or he imagined a wedge in his chest that could break through his bones. He imagined hearing the bones breaking open, splitting him like firewood. That's how he fell asleep at night.

While in the hospital, he'd kept a journal, and each entry started as a letter to Anne. He wanted to tell her everything that had happened over the years; how he felt about her, and how much he loved her. He wrote the letter, and then he wrote it again. He wrote one draft after another until he had hundreds of drafts, and he kept writing them, for years. When we spoke, he had eight years of drafts. But he never sent the letter.

Sometimes his mother sat next to him and cried.

In the hospital, when he couldn't leave, when the outside world vanished, the daydreams began. He craved intimacy with Anne so much that he'd try to create some semblance of it in fantasy.

He imagined she was asleep in the chair beside his bed. After lights out, when the nurses left, she woke up and emptied his liver bag, and then crawled into bed with him, and fell back asleep. She slept between his body and the rail.

In the dreams, if his mother cried, Anne was there to comfort her.

Mostly the dreams took on the landscape of the hospital, but there were also little dreams about camping and travel, about being on an airplane, traveling together—no tropical vacations—just going to see her family in Texas or his family in St. Louis. At night, once again, he liked to imagine that she helped him empty his liver bag. "I'll never leave you," she would tell him. "This is my fight too. I love you."

They did everything together in his dreams. He loved to imagine that slight but impactful feeling of her gripping his hand when he was least expecting it or them standing next to each other, feeling each other's heat. "Those small things that validate you as a human being," he said. "Because I've been searching for validation about the love that I think we had, or that I had for her, and in these daydreams, she lets me know that I am the person I'm supposed to be because that person is with her."

In the spring of 2015, the cancer was in remission and he was cast back into the world with no idea what to do. He chewed through his supply of OxyContin in six days, went through the agony of withdrawal on the couch. He bought pills on the streets, he checked himself into the ER for another bottle. He lived life three hours at a time, because that's how long the drug lasted before the pain began. The desire to get high was intense and gripping. Aaron compared it to the innate human desire to breed.

His cousin, an EMT worker, intervened by taking him out on a drive-along in Chicago to see the overdosed. Aaron promised to quit. In the morning, he searched for news of Anne and then regretted it. Someone else had found her first—she was engaged—the wedding date was a few months away. Not the news he wanted.

Without Anne, his thoughts again turned to suicide. He tried running again to make his heart explode, but he couldn't get it going fast enough. Weeks later, he learned the wedding was off. He took this as a sign, and it gave him enough motivation to pull himself out of depression. He took HTP supplements, L-tryptophan, antidepressants, and increased the number of miles he was running. In all these things, at their center was the belief that he could make Anne love him again.

We write a story for our lives, and we follow the story for a while, and then there is the life that we end up living. It was as if Aaron had written the ending to his fairy tale, but nothing he wrote got him to that end. "The daydreams will never stop," he told me, "and there will be new ones to come, and they make me feel something so special and it nourishes me. It's not a good supplement, but it's all I've got."

Aaron told me he'd given up on finding someone else. He wished things were different and that he could find happiness any other way. And he had tried. He tried to love two other women, but the intimacy with their bodies was strange. "People assume that I've built her up in my head, or made her into something that she's not. But I know enough about myself and I have enough of these stories to know that I don't look back on them and forget the bad parts and only remember the good."

Aaron hoped one day she would be in his arms again. Later, he admitted that if he were to meet Anne again, he wasn't sure how he would feel. Maybe he wouldn't want to meet her. She was better off a frozen woman, a sleeping beauty. Another corpse pulled from the river in France, propped in the morgue window.

"I've gotten really good at projecting whatever fantasy I have into reality," he told me. That's how he fell asleep at night, playing out scenarios in his head. "I can feel myself going into a trance, trying to imagine her."

In a dream—he's just finished a run and it's a five-hour

drive back, and the sun is turning to rain because he wants it that way. How much nicer it is to come home, wet and cold, to a warm bed? How incredible it will feel to come home to Anne while the rain blurs the windows! He gets back to his apartment, exhausted, and all he's going to do is sleep, the first good sleep he's had in years. Then she comes in and lies beside him, pulls the blanket over the both of them and falls alseep. "That is exactly where she wants to be," Aaron told me. "And nowhere else."

One Day at a Women's Prison

RACHEL WHITE-DOMAIN CRIED WHEN SHE SPOKE ABOUT THE women. "They are rotting in prison," she said.

We were at El Mazatlan, a Mexican restaurant across from the Super 8 in Lincoln, Illinois, eating fajitas and drinking beers with limes. Outside by the fountain, lightning bugs came around with their wings spread, looking like small angels. White-Domain was a public defender, trying to reduce the long prison sentences of mothers incarcerated for killing the men who were violent with them, acting in self-defense or in defense of their children. "If you want to see every facet of patriarchy," she told me, "spend one day in a women's prison." She was bare-faced and had tired but gentle eyes. Her hair was shoulder length and straight. I heard about White-Domain from the *Chicago Tribune*, how she was going to save women languishing in prisons. I found her because I wanted to know what happened to women who fought back. These were women who never got to tell their stories of self-defense. But now there was a small opportunity: In 2017, Illinois passed a law that gave women whose experiences of violence or abuse were not considered in their original sentencing a chance to tell their stories. The idea was that if people heard their stories of abuse and trauma, then the women wouldn't be locked up for half their lives, mothering children from afar. But when I showed up in Illinois, it was 2023, and most of the resentencing cases had failed. "If you are poor, and you are Black, and you are a woman," White-Domain told me, "it will be much harder."

It was the same process for all the women, and it took almost five years of interviews to get each story right. White-Domain shared the petitions with me before I arrived at the prison so that I would already know their stories. I saw photographs of the women from when they were children and photographs of when they were adults holding their own children. I read the children's letters, saying how much they wanted their moms back.

White-Domain always asked her clients to tell her the good things first, because the women wouldn't talk about the bad without first talking about the good. With grace, all the women told her about the people who hurt them. They loved their flawed mothers. They understood that their family or their partners had been through trauma that affected their ability to be present for them. There was a complexity to the way they saw the people in their lives who were either abusers or bystanders—complexities that sometimes made lawyers give up cases because of the way they told stories. They talked about loving an abuser or having a good childhood despite a catalog of horror. They didn't say, I'm a survivor and I know I did everything right. They didn't tell their stories like that.

At the restaurant that evening, White-Domain told me that part of her job meant listening to the recorded calls the women made from prison. And she had listened to all 250 calls made by her client Debraca Harris, and all of them were with her kids, helping them with math homework, telling them not to drink Pepsi. "Just being a good mother," she said. Debraca talked to her kids every day. They got twenty minutes on the phone, and then they had to wait thirty or thirty-five minutes to get back on.

The news usually made these women look like cold-blooded murderers who killed men over microwaves, or disputes about the bills. They were portrayed as women who were doing just fine until one day, out of nowhere, they "snapped."

When White-Domain picked me up the next morning, she asked if I could bring tissues. I didn't know why until I got in her car. Is it for the crying? I asked. She nodded.

Logan Correctional Center is the largest women's prison in Illinois. It was the end of May and everything was blooming. Insects flew in and out of the tall wire fences to pollinate the prison's small gardens. Women walked around unchained, wearing uniforms of white shirts and navy pants or shorts. A row of leafy sycamore grew tall out of the parking lot. Clouds with glowing edges and dark centers gathered in the sky. Gunshots rang out from the cornfields. "That always happens," White-Domain told me. "The women are always complaining."

The facility looked more like an elementary school than a prison, with about a dozen low redbrick buildings with black shingled roofs, walking paths through mown lawn, and gardens. Barbed wire sagged around paint-chipped guard towers. It didn't look like it would be that hard to escape.

The unsmiling faces of mothers on mood-altering drugs turned to stare as we walked past.

The creaky building we entered was full of muted light and worn wood furniture. It smelled musty. We were patted down, checked for weapons, and scanned for paraphernalia.

A guard took us in one building and out another, past a sign that warned inmates that they'd be shot if they approached an aircraft. The guard showed us to a windowless room with cracked linoleum floors. There was a broken clock on the wall, and, in the corner, something that looked like a confessional with a little smeared window.

We were here to talk to Debraca Harris and Antheshia "Angel" Lee, both charged with first-degree murder committed in acts of self-defense. Later, we would visit Laconda McDonald at Decatur Correctional Center, a thirty-minute drive away.

Debraca Harris showed up first. She was soft-spoken and petite, with her hair slicked back in a ballerina bun, lips shaped like a heart. She wore a light gray T-shirt with knee-length navy shorts. Debraca was forty-four and the mother of five children. She worked at the prison beauty salon. In 2006, her landlord sexually assaulted her and punched her in the face as he handed over an eviction notice. He'd been trying to rape her, and said he'd give her free rent if she consented. Debraca shot him.

Angel arrived late, with her dreads pulled back into a ponytail, high and loose. There was a little white cowrie shell in one of the strands. Her hazel eyes were framed with a shimmer of translucent shadow. She was a mother who had been sexually harassed and stalked by a drug dealer. She stabbed the man in the parking lot of a 7-Eleven after he hit her in the face. She was forty-one and stood five foot two, the same height as Debraca.

The prison trusted them enough to let them take care of themselves. They trusted Debraca enough to hold scissors when she worked as a hairdresser. These were rehabilitated women, no longer the traumatized mothers they were years ago.

A guard slumped in a desk chair outside the door and listened.

Angel pointed to the guard. "Does he need to be here?" We

all nodded. "I just know they gossip about our personal stuff," she said. "I don't like it, but it is what it is."

There was no air-conditioning. It was eighty-five degrees outside and the air was heavy. The guard let Angel grab a dust-coated plastic fan. It spun hot air in our faces.

Debraca smiled. "My energy's a little calmer than hers," she said of Angel. "She's up every morning doing workouts. She's a pistol." Angel used to run track. She was long-legged and quick.

When it came time to talk, Angel said, "We already told our stories." She crossed her arms. Debraca said the same. "We told Rachel our stories for five years. Nothing changed."

"Well, maybe that's the story," White-Domain said.

Even if no one listened to their stories now, she added, maybe one day they would, and people would hear the stories and they would say how they couldn't believe anyone was ever treated the way Debraca and Angel were treated. "The same way we talk about slavery or the witch trials," White-Domain said. "That kind of thing."

The women shrugged. If one day someone cared, maybe that was enough.

White-Domain pulled out some loose tissues she had stashed in her purse and set them on the table. They were wrinkled but clean.

They were not easy stories to hear, but these were the lives these women had lived.

Debraca's Story

Debraca told me she was the kind of person who, if she was called beautiful, would be polite and say thank you. But she would never believe you.

Debraca started running away when she was thirteen, but didn't tell anyone why. She was taught that you weren't supposed to talk about the bad things. You certainly didn't talk about your stepdad's sexual abuse. You didn't tell your friends and you didn't tell your teacher. You didn't tell your aunt and you certainly didn't tell the Chicago police, who had been known for literally torturing dozens of Black men for over thirty years. She wasn't going to do that. And Debraca didn't want to hurt her mother. She knew her stepdad was the reason her mother didn't have to struggle anymore. If her mother left him, they'd be broke again and back to living in the projects on Chicago's East Side, worrying about the electricity going off, worrying about hunger. Debraca told me her favorite part of elementary school was that she got to eat lunch.

So she started running away to her dad's house. He was addicted to crack, but she felt safe with him. When she was fourteen and living with her dad, a friend invited her over to hang out at her house, and the friend's boyfriend locked Debraca in a bedroom and wouldn't let her leave. She was kept there for two days and forced to have sex with different men. She kept this a secret too. It was her first sexual experience besides her stepdad. When friends at school found out, they called her a slut.

After that she was running away all the time to have sex with older boys in the neighborhood because they gave her a place to stay and they gave her the attention she wanted. The kind of attention that sometimes felt like love. In high school, she remembered herself as "a young woman looking for someone to love her for who she was." She was looking for the hugs and the kisses, and she longed to hear "You're beautiful" or "You're appreciated," but she usually got the opposite. If she slept with a guy and he didn't care about her, she told herself she could deal. But after a while it wore her down.

When Debraca got pregnant at fifteen, she kept it a secret until she couldn't. She didn't want an abortion, but her mom forced her to have one. It was a three-day event: feticide, intact dilation, evacuation, follow-up. It was traumatic for her. That baby was, at six months, almost formed. Someone she wanted. Someone who might love her.

When she and her mom got in fights, an older guy named Jason would come over and get her and they would stay at Jason's mom's house. Because of what happened with her step-dad, she never really wanted to be at her mom's house. She thought Jason would protect her. Jason got her pregnant, and this time her mother let Debraca keep it. Debraca was eighteen and had a high school diploma, and her mother said the decision was hers. She was happy until she found out there was another girl who was pregnant with Jason's baby at the same time. Debraca was devastated.

She believed Jason loved her, but he had women all over the place. He wasn't the settling-down type, and Debraca wanted a father for her kids.

Debraca enrolled in Dudley Beauty College in a cinder-block building on Chicago's South Side to learn haircutting. Inside were mannequin heads she used to braid, brush, cut, style, spray. They did nails, long press-on nails with bling, glitter, wings of every color and length. She loved it. It's what she always wanted to do. When she was in sixth grade, she'd started experimenting with hair. That's what she would do with her friends. They would come over to her house and they would listen to music and she would do their hair. She was working to get her degree all through her pregnancy. She had this whole plan in her head. If she kept working, she would have the license before she had the baby.

But Debraca was scared. She didn't want to have to raise this baby by herself, and she didn't want to be at her mother's house either because of her stepdad. She had no resources and nowhere to go. So when she reconnected with Willie Collins, she had a lot of hope. He was a year older. They went to the same middle school and lived in the same neighborhood growing up. It was like she already knew him. She knew him as a friend. He was familiar. She was eight months pregnant, but he accepted her. She wanted her baby to have a father. She was gone all day at beauty school working hard. She would start at eight in the morning and wouldn't leave the building until eight in the evening. But Willie didn't like that she was gone all day. You're pregnant and you're on your feet all day, he told her. You don't need to be doing that.

So she quit beauty school.

After Debraca gave birth, Willie left her.

When the baby was about two weeks old, and Willie was long gone, Debraca started to feel strange, agitated, and overwhelmed. The baby cried and she felt helpless. Sometimes she became frozen, dissociated, and nonresponsive. Her mother noticed Debraca wanted to sleep all the time. On a difficult day when the baby was crying, Debraca had an urge to shake her, and this disturbed Debraca, so she put the baby in her mother's care and left the house. She was overwhelmed, never screened for postpartum depression or given support.

After that, desperate for money and independence, Debraca started stripping. It was just a means to an end. She was trying to get out of her mom's house.

Then she was pregnant again. The father was a man she met at the strip club, and they'd been on a couple of dates. She was having a boy, and she really wanted the man at the club to be in this baby's life. But when he found out she was pregnant, he just stopped talking to her, he just disappeared. He didn't want to be around. He had other kids.

Now she was a single mother with two kids and neither one of their dads around. "It was painful," she told me. "Because you judge yourself."

Around this time, Debraca attempted suicide, and woke up in the emergency room.

Debraca started dating Willie again when she was twenty-three. She felt lucky he wanted to be with her even though she had these two children with other fathers. At the time Willie worked at a factory, and he provided for them. She also liked his mother, Helen, and his family accepted her. Finally, Debraca thought, I have a protector and I'm okay.

"Then, when I got pregnant with our first kid, Willie flipped. It was like: Now you're pregnant with mine. He could control me."

After Willie became violent and pushed her pregnant body down the stairs, she fled in the middle of the night on a Greyhound bound for Atlanta. It was where her family had relocated. Away from Willie's abuse, and with her mom and sister's support, she got a job as the manager of a title loan company and moved into her own apartment. In July 2003, when the baby was born, she looked into her little girl's eyes and knew she was never going to get away from Willie. She was unable to feel any joy or pleasure. Every baby left her with postpartum depression without her knowing what that was.

Willie insisted on flying down to see the baby because it was his firstborn—he made Debraca feel guilty for keeping the child away from him. After Willie got to Atlanta, he promised he would change and pressured Debraca to move back to Illinois with him. She gave up her life in Atlanta and moved back with Willie to Harvey, Illinois.

Debraca's mother kept a house in Harvey that she'd been renting out, and Debraca and Willie moved in there. The monthly mortgage on the house was $1,200, but with so many kids she couldn't pay. Willie got frustrated even though he didn't have a job either. He would take it out on her. "And it wasn't like I could go to anybody to ask for help," she said.

Four months after giving birth, she got pregnant again. This child was born in the summer of 2004, thirteen months after her last child was born. Debraca was now twenty-five and had four children under the age of seven. This was around the time when the black eyes and busted lips started. Whether she was pregnant or not, Willie didn't care. He would work out at the boxing gym and use what he learned on Debraca. He strangled her until she passed out. He would punch her so much that she would just roll up into a ball on the floor. Soon he started beating just her body, not her face, so that no one would see the bruises.

Willie's mother, Helen, asked Debraca, "Why don't you leave him?" Debraca started crying. She just wanted the kids to have a father. "Because I love them so much," she said.

Helen could see the sadness in Debraca even when she tried to hide it.

Willie would hurt Debraca, she'd leave for a few days, then he'd get calm and say he needed her, and she'd return.

When Debraca had no money to feed her kids or herself, they went to a grocery store and just started eating food in the store. They were in a state of severe poverty and housing insta-bility. And Willie was the most violent when the bills were due.

It was late 2005, and she was five months pregnant with her fifth child. She was twenty-six years old and she had no energy left to care for another child. Sometimes, Debraca wondered if Willie wanted to keep her pregnant to control her because all of the pregnancies were back-to-back.

After they defaulted on the mortgage at Debraca's mother's home, Willie went to stay with his mom, and Debraca went to stay with her cousin Lynn.

Debraca's oldest daughter was tired of moving and begged Debraca to "please find [them] a home." Debraca wanted to give her children some normalcy instead of dragging them around to different people's houses. They had been moving in circles. They moved between the houses of cousins and the spare bedrooms of friends. Usually they would just move instead of paying rent because they didn't have the money. Debraca was done waiting for Willie to help them. And after ten years together, she really wasn't looking for his support anymore anyway. So when Debraca saw a FOR RENT sign outside a small home with a lawn, she called the number. The landlord's name was Tracy Jones, and he didn't ask too many questions. He didn't care that Debraca was unemployed. Debraca signed the lease that day and she, Willie, and the kids moved in. Debraca knew she would have trouble paying rent, but she just needed to put a roof over her kids' heads. She paid the first month's rent with public assistance and prayed she'd figure out the rest.

When the next month came around, and she didn't have the money, she called the landlord to ask for more time and expected him to start yelling. She was surprised when he spoke in a calm voice and told her she could give him "sexual services" in exchange for rent. He said it just like that—"sexual services"—as if it were official business. The idea disgusted her, but this was her chance to give her children a real home. She would do anything for them. She was tired of bouncing around, and she was going to do whatever she had to do to keep her kids off the street and to keep Willie from beating her. If she had to sacrifice her body, then she was going to do it. "I brought them into the world," she told me. "They didn't ask to be here. So how could I let them down?"

The landlord's assaults happened during Debraca's sixth, seventh, eighth, and ninth months of pregnancy. The sex was rough, painful, and humiliating. She was bleeding and swollen. When she begged for the landlord to end the sex-for-rent arrangement, he threatened to tell Willie that they were having an affair. She knew what Willie would do to her—he might kill her—so she kept meeting with the landlord. They met in parking lots, alleys, side streets, or dingy hotels. He had a green car and a white car. He always demanded oral sex first. He threatened her with eviction over and over again. The landlord never told Debraca anything about himself and never asked anything about Debraca either. When she was nine months pregnant, she cried and worried he was hurting her baby. It didn't seem to bother him the way it bothered her. She would cry, but he wasn't moved by her tears or her pleading. To cope, she repeated in her head: My kids can go home. Me and the kids are going home.

After she gave birth to her fifth child, she decided she couldn't take it anymore. She was done and he could kick them out. During this time Debraca felt absent from her life. She didn't have words for what was going on—she didn't have time for words. She was tired in a way that made her body feel like it wasn't there. Sometimes she would be taking care of her baby and she would feel herself sucked back into the landlord's arms. She did not bond with the baby. She barely looked at the baby. She did not want to touch the baby. Each day, she got the kids ready for school and took them to school and picked them up from school. She made sure they ate. She made sure Willie was okay. She skipped meals to make sure her kids had enough food. Survive, survive, survive, she repeated. The kids were all that kept her going. These little creatures that depended on her. They were the only reason she smiled.

The landlord called her on the sixth of June to remind Debraca she needed to be out. She was still packing things in the car and she hadn't told Willie yet about the eviction, because she didn't want to deal with him. The landlord kept calling and bothering her about restarting their agreement and she told him no, but that she would meet him one more time to try to negotiate. Since she wasn't going to have sex with him, she didn't think it would be a problem. Before she left the house, she packed up a few more things. She wasn't sure if the landlord would let her back in, so she grabbed Willie's gun and put it in the diaper bag.

They met in an alley and Debraca got in the landlord's car. The baby was in a carrier and she put the carrier in the back seat. The landlord said, "Let's go to a hotel." She said, "I've got my baby. I can't do it. I can't do it." He grabbed her and she pushed him off. He yanked her head into his lap for a blow job and she pushed him off again. She got her baby out of his back seat and ran back to her car. While she was getting her baby buckled, the landlord called her name. He said he had something to give her, and Debraca wondered if he had changed his mind. She went to his driver's-side window, and he handed her a piece of paper and told her again that she had to be out of the house. "Please," she said. "Get in the car," he said. He reached through the window, grabbed her shirt, and punched her in the face. Debraca grabbed the gun and shot him.

"Or I shot someone who looked like him because the face I saw was also Willie's face," she said. "It was like the two men had morphed into one face."

On the day of her arrest, Debraca was still bleeding. The police brought all five kids with her to the station, and then brought them back home. She didn't know that the landlord was dead. When they told her she killed him, she replied that she ought to kill herself.

"It appears she was having an affair with him," Sandra Alvarado, a spokeswoman for the Harvey Police Department, told the *Chicago Tribune* in June 2006.

Debraca woke up the next day chained to a hospital bed and had no memory of talking to the police. A public defender stopped by and told Debraca where she shot the landlord—point-blank in the head.

"I didn't do that," she said.

"Yes, you did."

"I did it there?"

She didn't know what kind of gun it was; she just knew it was black.

She was medicated and kept in a single padded cell of the Cook County Jail psych unit. They kept her there because she wasn't talking and she wasn't moving much either. She spent six months there until the meds started working and she started remembering the landlord's bloodshot eyes. She didn't mean to kill him.

Cook County Jail is the largest in the country, about the size of seventy-two football fields. Most everyone inside was like her—African Americans or Latinos from Chicago's South and West Sides who'd been charged with murder. It was designed to be a temporary place, but it didn't always work that way. Debraca waited six years.

At the courthouse in 2012, Debraca had been prepared to tell her story of self-defense. Her whole family was there. But the state offered her a plea deal: thirty years in exchange for a guilty plea. Debraca's attorney told her that if she didn't take the plea deal, she would get sixty years.

"I'm oblivious to the law. I don't know what's going on. And I'm trusting this man that they've hired to represent me. And he's telling me that I'm going to get sixty years, and I'm comparing that to thirty. So I'm like, well, can I talk to my family? And he said no, we don't have enough time for that. So I said, okay, just give me the plea deal. And that's when I took the thirty years."

When the attorneys discussed the plea deal, they weren't required to say anything about Debraca's life—they only needed to give enough facts for the judge to convict. It's a couple of sentences, and in cases involving self-defense, it usually just says that somebody was shot and killed. And that's what happened in Debraca's case. She never had the chance to bring up the full extent of the abuse she suffered from her boyfriend or her landlord.

Debraca was a rape victim who acted in self-defense but entered the Illinois Department of Corrections with a thirty-year sentence to be served at 100 percent for first-degree murder. She never met with domestic-violence experts. She wasn't evaluated by a postpartum expert or a rape advocate.

Debraca went to the Illinois Penitentiary for Women at Dwight, an hour south of Chicago, and it was rough. She got in trouble because she had to learn the rules: when to shower, when to turn off the lights, when to eat. She wore a red badge that signaled she was the kind of prisoner you needed to watch out for. She spent her whole life being abused, and now people looked at her as if she were the dangerous one. At night, she was quiet when she cried.

At the same time, prison was the first place she had ever lived without having violence done to her body. It was strange for her. She took a little extra time in the shower and she always made sure her clothes looked nice. She started reading books, sewing, drawing, and painting, and she never knew she liked any of these things. She discovered all these things that she was good at, and she even started to like herself.

But Debraca didn't get to see her newborn until he was about a year old.

"You got to hold him?" I asked.

"No," she said. "It was through the glass."

Debraca was never given a chance at parole or the opportunity for a mid-sentence review. Legally there was no way for Debraca to tell her story of self-defense. Ten years passed before Rachel White-Domain walked into Logan Correctional Center and asked to represent Debraca. Illinois had just introduced a new law that allowed lawyers to petition for more lenient sentences for domestic-abuse and sexual-assault survivors.

It took a whole team of people to tell Debraca's story—lawyers, psychologists, victim advocates, postpartum experts, law students. They gathered medical records, orders of protection, time spent in domestic-violence shelters. They combed over her entire life. They gathered affidavits from her sisters, mother, extended family, and sometimes from ex-boyfriends admitting to abuse and regretting it. White-Domain made copies of every certificate earned in prison, every class and degree, as well as violations. Social workers wrote letters attesting to Debraca's plans for reintegration.

Five years later, in December 2017, when White-Domain finished Debraca's petition for resentencing, it was one hundred and eighty pages long. She offered the state's attorney a copy to read, and the state's attorney still didn't believe Debraca was a rape victim. She believed the sex was consensual—that it was a sex-for-rent situation.

"I was blown away," White-Domain told me. "To be clear, she wasn't saying, 'I don't think that happened.' The words she said to me were, 'I don't see her as a rape victim because I see that as a consensual exchange.'"

In April 2020, during a three-day hearing, White-Domain fought to reduce Debraca's sentence from thirty years to twenty years. The judge agreed with all the evidence White-Domain presented: that Debraca Harris was a mother who suffered abuse and sexual assault by her partner and by her landlord, and that the landlord had threatened her with eviction in exchange for sex. The judge agreed she was severely traumatized and acting on survival instincts. Despite all this, her sentence was reduced by only three years.

"The judge literally, on the record," White-Domain told me, "made a finding, 'Yes, I believe you. How about twenty-seven years instead of thirty?' So what's the win there?"

The resentencing law was written so that a judge could learn that Debraca was a survivor of domestic and sexual violence who acted in self-defense. She was dragged through three days of retelling on top of years and years of retelling the same story. "The takeaway," White-Domain said, "isn't that we need more laws that say we should have believed them. Because it's not going to mean they don't end up spending the rest of their life in prison. And it probably won't even mean that they're going to get a shorter sentence. A judge could believe her all day. A judge could believe every single word that came out of her mouth. And he, more or less, said that he did."

After the judge's decision, White-Domain said her colleague, Alexis Mansfield, an expert in incarcerated women, asked, "Is it worse when they don't believe you? Or is it worse when they believe you, but it doesn't matter?"

Angel's Story

When Angel told her family about her uncle's sexual abuse, her grandmother took her to a prophet. The prophet put his hand on the Bible, and her grandmother asked if Angel's story was true, and the prophet said, "Yeah, that happened," and Angel was like, "I told you so." They went to Ace Hardware and Angel's grandmother said, "Don't tell anybody. We are not talking about this."

To escape her uncle, Angel was almost never home, and that's how she started dating Todd, who lived down the street. Angel was sixteen and Todd was twenty-seven. Todd bought Angel everything a sixteen-year-old girl could ever want. Six months after she moved in with him she was pregnant, and because she was pregnant, Todd told her she didn't need to leave the house. When she was allowed out occasionally, he started checking her panties every time she returned home to make sure she wasn't cheating. To her, it felt like a small price to pay considering all he had done for her. And Angel thought it was his way of showing he cared.

One time Angel was at the hairdresser and Todd was ready

to pick her up. Todd always picked her up and dropped her off, but this time she wanted to take the bus and visit a friend to watch a movie and eat snacks from the gas station. Todd showed up, banging on the door. He was furious. He took her outside, grabbed her hair, and slammed her head on the asphalt. Angel saw his eyes turn black. He dragged her body through the alleyway. He pushed her down and then made her get back up. When they got back to the house, he told her, "Bitch, I'm going to lock you in this room with bread and water. You're only getting out to go to the bathroom." And she didn't even have words. She was just crying because she thought Todd was the one who was going to protect her. He checked her underwear. She cried until he started crying too. "I'm sorry," he said, "you just make me so crazy. I love you, I love you." And she thought: Maybe he does love me? Maybe he doesn't know how to express it? And then she started feeling like she was the problem, and if she could just do the right things then she could help him do right too. Todd was good at telling Angel exactly what she needed to hear. The things she had always wished somebody would've said to her. He said, "I need you. I want you. I love you."

But he didn't change. Todd checked Angel's panties again every time she failed to check in on time, or if he didn't know where she was during the day.

One night a friend called and told Angel she had a place for her to stay in DeKalb, a small town an hour west of Chicago. Angel took her daughter and left that night.

In Dekalb, Angel got a job as a cashier at Amoco Super Pantry and started classes at the local college. She wanted to take a break from men but was drawn to twenty-three-year-old Vernon Washington, who treated her well and never beat her.

They moved in together to save money, splitting the rent with Vernon's cousin Lamar. Vernon grew up poor and was dealing drugs to help support his mother and father. He had this little clique of dealers who Angel thought were shabby and dirty, and she told Vernon to quit them and get a degree. Vernon planned on it but was having trouble with rent, so he wanted to make one more deal before he quit. That one deal got him locked up, and while he was locked up, a new guy came onto the scene and linked up with Vernon's crew. His name was Antonio "Tony" Cureton, and he was handsome and dressed like he had a lot of money. One day Angel's car engine locked up and she had no way to see Vernon in jail, so Lamar asked Tony to take them.

Angel had never met Tony, and when she got in the back seat, he stared hard at her through the rearview mirror. He asked her name and she said, "Angel." He asked if she had ever cheated on Vernon and she said she hadn't. He said he thought he could make her cheat and she said she doubted it. He said he only messed with "queens," and the fact that he was even talking to her should make her feel lucky. She said she didn't care. He said she had a smart-ass mouth. She said you don't have to talk. He called her a bitch and said she could get out and walk. Lamar told Angel to stop. They were on a dirt road in the middle of nowhere on the way to Sycamore, Illinois, to get to the jail. She rolled in silence the rest of the way. When the trip was over, Tony told Angel she needed to think about her attitude. She got out, closed the door, and left.

Tony started making his drug crew more money than Vernon ever did, and their loyalty turned to him.

Angel didn't see Tony again until Lamar brought him over to their apartment. They were going to a concert, and Lamar needed to shower and get dressed before they left. "Can he just come in and sit in the living room?" Lamar asked. And he apologized for Tony's behavior in the car and said he thought he was just high or something. Angel said it was okay, and Tony came into the living room while Lamar took a shower.

Angel sat on the couch wearing stretch pants and a white tank top and put her legs up on a chair. Tony looked out the blinds behind the couch, then looked at her. "You have a phat-ass pussy," he said. "Is it as good as it looks? Can I ask your boy Vernon?"

Angel jumped up and knocked on the bathroom door, where Lamar was still taking his shower. "He has to go," she said. "Get him out of here."

Tony called her uptight and said he had no problem hitting women and that, in fact, he had hit a lady police officer a couple years back. He said the same would happen to her if she continued to act tough by rejecting his advances.

Angel couldn't get Tony to leave her alone. It became a pattern she couldn't escape. Everywhere she went, he found her and made comments about her sexy body.

Vernon got out of jail in early March 2001, and on the night of March thirtieth two members of Tony's crew came to Vernon and Angel's apartment claiming to be from the DeKalb Police Department. It was Jaymo and Big Country, and the two of them pistol-whipped Vernon in the face, pushed their way inside, tied up Vernon and Lamar, and robbed them of their phones, IDs, and two eight balls of crack. Angel was out of town with her daughter, but they went into her room and arranged all her thongs and negligees on the floor like a warning.

Vernon was at the hospital when he called Angel to tell

her what happened. They must have expected her to have been home. "They were definitely going to rape me," she told him, "and then they were going to have to kill me because my daughter would've been there with me."

After that, she always carried a knife.

A month later, seven of Tony's crew showed up at Burritoville where Angel, Vernon, and their friend Syndana were eating lunch. Angel immediately called the police. Vernon and the crew started arguing, and Angel yelled for them to stop. One of the men punched Vernon in the face. Syndana began pleading for someone to help. Then one of the crew members punched Syndana and Angel pulled out the knife. The man punching Syndana stopped and backed out of the restaurant. When the police arrived, they saw Angel with the knife in her hand. She dropped the knife and tried to explain what was happening, including that she was the one who called 911, but they arrested her.

Syndana remembered that one or more of the men said they were going to "put Angel in the trunk" and kidnap her. Angel, who had never been arrested before, was given bond and left the county jail after just a few days. When she returned home, a brick had been thrown through the balcony window of her apartment. The DeKalb *Daily Chronicle* wrote that Angel was "charged with aggravated battery and mob action after she allegedly threatened to kill an unnamed victim inside of the restaurant."

Angel kept seeing Tony around. He was at a concert, at the Walmart parking lot, at the tire shop, always calling her name and yelling jokes about Vernon.

About a week later, Angel was with her friend Ant at the 7-Eleven behind her apartment building, buying cigarettes.

They saw Tony in the parking lot. She didn't want to talk to him and she walked away. "Why you gotta walk away from me?" he yelled out the window of his blue Oldsmobile. "You mad about what happened to your boyfriend?" He was going on and on and on.

She said she didn't have time for this. She turned around and walked away again. He touched her arm and she recoiled. Ant tried to stop them from fighting but backed away. Angel told Tony not to touch her. She tried walking away from the situation three times, and when she refused to pacify him, he lost his patience and "muffed" her, meaning that he thrust his whole hand over her face and shoved her back hard enough that she "stumbled backward," not just one but a "couple steps." Then Tony raised a clenched fist over her head. She turned her head away from his fist, grabbed the knife in her pocket, and held it in front of her face. She didn't know she had stabbed him until Tony put his hands on his chest and she saw blood. He was still alive when she left. He was still coming after her.

Tony leaned against the wall of the 7-Eleven and held his wound. He stood there for a minute before he slowly slid down the wall.

Angel went into her apartment, sat her purse down, and lit a cigarette.

She did not know he was dead until hours after she was taken to the police station. It was May 2001. The knife hit an artery and he bled internally. But what the medical examiner later explained was that the force was consistent with Tony's falling into the knife.

Angel went to trial, and was convicted of first-degree murder and sentenced to twenty-nine years. She was nineteen at the time of her arrest.

White-Domain spent five years working on Angel's two-hundred-page petition. She argued that Angel was a victim of "male-on-female rejection violence."

When White-Domain submitted the petition after five years of interviews and evidence collection, the judges called the petition "untimely and without merit."

Laconda's Story

I heard Laconda McDonald before I saw her. She was in the hallway without cuffs, wearing sweatpants and a sweatshirt. She walked slowly with aching knees, all three hundred pounds of her. "Hot Girl" was tattooed on her right arm, and "Death Before Love" on her left. The names of boyfriends and pimps were tattooed all over her body: Mike, Andre, Eddie, J.B.

She had high round cheeks, a round nose, and a large mouth with a thin upper lip. Her eyes were deep set and dark, almost blue around the edges. She had bangs and styled her hair somewhere between a mullet and a bowl cut.

"I'm tired of telling my story over and over again," Laconda told me. "I've told my story and nothing happened."

She already told her family and her lawyers, and nothing changed. She told the *Chicago Tribune* and nothing changed. She was in a documentary about incarcerated victims and they quoted her and nothing changed. Then she told White-Domain her story, which took five years of retelling, and nothing changed. Her resentencing petition was denied; her clemency petition was denied.

Laconda's attorney, Susan Smith, had tried to get Laconda to go to trial because she thought she could argue self-defense. But Laconda had lived her whole life not being believed, and she didn't want to be humiliated on the witness stand. Everything she had been told about herself played in her head: You're ugly, you're a crackhead, you're a prostitute, and you're Black. So why even fight? By then she'd already spent a month in jail and didn't want to drag it out. She didn't want to relive that day again. She thought she should get those twenty years because that's what the state's attorney told her she deserved.

On November 13, 2012, Laconda was sentenced to twenty years in prison for first-degree murder, to be served at 100 percent.

Had Laconda gone to trial and been convicted of murder in the second degree, she would have already served her time, even if she received the maximum penalty under the law.

"I could tell my story," she told me, "but why? I'm here in prison, alone, feeling unloved, unwanted, going through what I'm going through. Mistreated, abused, called fat and ugly again. It's getting tedious. What's the sense of me telling the same story over and over again? Nothing changes. Nobody cares. They say, oh it's a Black girl, a crackhead, a prostitute. She should have left that man. That's how they see it. Nothing changes, nothing good comes from me telling the same story. Right after this, guess what? I'm going to go back to my cell and I'm going to be sad." Laconda lifted her arm and rolled up her sleeve. "He bit me here," she told me. "That is a human bite." There it was. A human bite from Julius Goodman. The scar tissue had risen up smooth and round to form what looked like a pair of lips.

Laconda's stepfather's abuse started when she was eight years old. Laconda told her mother about it, but her mother didn't believe her. She believed him. Her stepfather threatened to hurt her mother and kill her family if Laconda mentioned it again. "And I loved my Mama. I didn't want nothing happening to my Mama."

Most days they didn't have much food to eat. They had places to live sometimes and other times they didn't. One home was an unfinished apartment with just a sink and a toilet with no bath or hot water. Sometimes they lived in shelters or on couches. Sometimes with an uncle or a grandmother. They got food stamps that were supposed to last a month but really lasted two weeks. They would sleep in one room with the sheets up over the windows, trying to stay warm. At Christmas, there were no presents. Her mother lied and said it was because Laconda was "bad" and Santa Claus was going to throw ash in her eyes. Laconda only wore donated clothes from church that sometimes got a wash on the weekends and sometimes didn't. She tried but she couldn't hide the poverty. She was poorer than the other poor kids. The Humboldt Park neighborhood of Chicago was a predominantly Spanish area, and she was bullied for being dark. They called her dirty. One time when she was sitting alone in the lunchroom, a kid poured a carton of chocolate milk on her face and everyone laughed. Another kid told her, "You have fleas on your face," and pretended to flick the fleas away. After school the kids beat her. Nobody at home told Laconda she was beautiful or other things that she wanted to hear. So she went home after school and listened to Prince's "Purple Rain" and looked at herself in the mirror and repeated: You are beautiful, you are beautiful, you are beautiful.

She started running away when she was twelve. She did what she needed to do to feed herself, and when she was just thirteen, she learned she was pregnant. One of her teachers cried when he found out. She finished the eighth grade and then dropped out. At first she didn't know who the father was, whether it was her stepfather or her boyfriend, a neighborhood kid called Cabbage, and when she found out it was her boyfriend, she left home for good.

The baby, a little girl, was born five days before Laconda's fourteenth birthday. She moved onto the streets with her newborn, staying sometimes with friends, sometimes with Carter, a sixteen-year-old, who introduced her to crack. She did crack because she wanted to be cool and she wanted him to like her. He called her ugly and threw food in her face if she didn't cook for him. When she got pregnant again, he kicked her out of the house so he could have sex with another woman. Laconda didn't have anywhere to go so she just slept on the porch while they had sex.

By the time she was sixteen she had two babies with Carter, in addition to the baby she had with Cabbage, and now she was addicted to crack. Those years she would only go home to ask her mom for three things: money to buy drugs, help taking care of a new baby, or permission to get her tubes tied.

Every time Laconda had a baby, she handed it over to her mother. Her mother tried to raise them all until social services showed up to find all these babies but no electricity, no cooking gas, and no food in the kitchen except popcorn. And that was around the time Laconda's mother started to wrap curtains around her head and talk in a strange language about Christ. Laconda and her siblings didn't know any better until she got a diagnosis for schizophrenia years too late.

Laconda was still a child. She was homeless and living on the streets, consumed by addiction. She worried about where she was going to sleep, what she was going to eat, and where she was going to take a shower. Sometimes she'd steal food to eat so as not to starve. One time she ate food out of the garbage—that's how hungry she was. Sometimes she used to go wash up in McDonald's or White Castle. ("Because a woman should not be on the street without taking a shower," she told me. "It's not a good thing. Oh, Lord, it's not a good thing.") Sometimes she slept at Cook County Hospital ("where you can go and just act like you're seeing a doctor"). She did that a lot. Sometimes she was so cold she would sign herself into a mental hospital and stay there until she was warm again. In the summer, she'd go to the third floor of a building where it was cool and she'd sleep on a piece of cardboard.

She starting doing sex work to feed herself. Often she was violently assaulted by her clients. It was lonely work on the streets and the most dangerous kind—where you can't screen clients and you rely on them to give you the place to have sex—their car or their house. It might be isolated and no one can hear you scream. A lot of bad things happened after two in the morning. Every time she got in a car, she cried.

In 1995, when Laconda was seventeen, she started a relationship with Charles, who forced himself into the role of her pimp. He was not good to her. Once, he locked Laconda in the basement for two months so that she wouldn't go do things without him. He made Laconda urinate in a hole in the floor.

When she got pregnant, he denied that it was his baby and kept saying that it was the mailman's baby. She had to keep selling her body because he wouldn't support her financially. He threw a forty-ounce beer bottle at the back of her head. Two weeks after she turned eighteen she gave birth to her fourth child. In July 1998, when she was twenty-one, Laconda gave birth to a daughter. Nine months later she gave birth to twin boys, Joshua and Jonathan. The father of the twins was unknown because it was someone she met for sex work.

She met another pimp named Andre while buying drugs. One time he punched Laconda and told her, "Okay, you can leave me now." And Laconda told him, "I will never leave you because I love you." That's how badly Laconda wanted love.

She made ten, twenty, thirty, forty dollars a date and would need about five or six dates a night to make enough money to keep Andre from hurting her. Sometimes she made a hundred dollars if the men felt sorry for her.

In her early twenties, Laconda had a breakdown. At this point, she was completely unable to function and felt like her brain did not work like everyone else's. She started hearing voices from her past repeating the mean things that people used to say to her. Over the next several months and years, on various occasions, she was admitted to St. Anthony's, St. Mary's, and St. Elizabeth's hospitals in Chicago. In 1999, when Laconda was twenty-two, she was institutionalized at Westshire Nursing & Rehabilitation Center in Cicero, Illinois, where she stayed for over a year with the help of disability benefits. Laconda thought it was a respite from her life. She got sober, began a medication regimen, and got some insight as to how her past trauma was affecting her substance use. When she got out, she had nowhere to go, so she went back to the house of her ex-pimp Charles. It was a drug house. Charles wasn't even there because he was in jail. She started smoking crack again.

It was 2001, and Laconda was on the winter streets with cold feet, when a man named Julius rolled by. He was five foot five and bald, with a mustache. He told her to get in the car, and she got in. The car was so warm and comfortable that she started crying. He took her home. She was about twenty-four and he was forty-six. She was waiting for him to try to have sex with her, but he told her not to worry, they didn't need to have sex. No one had ever said that to Laconda. Not ever.

In the shower, she closed her eyes and felt her muscles go from stiff to loose. Later she cooked dinner for the both of them—chicken and rice with corn—and they talked about her childhood. She told funny jokes and they laughed together, even about the things that weren't funny. His bed was so soft she called it "freaky." It didn't take much to keep her. "I gave him that power right there," she said.

The next night, Julius spooned Laconda, and she had never been spooned. Even with her children's fathers—it was always just sex with them. It felt like he truly wanted to be with her.

———

For the next ten years Laconda would remember those two nights and hoped for more of them, but Julius did not give Laconda the love she dreamed about.

Julius was addicted to cocaine and his drug habit got worse and worse. Men started coming over because Julius was bringing them to the house and asking Laconda to have sex with them. They paid Julius directly. She didn't see any money. Laconda didn't use the words "sex trafficking," but that's what was happening.

About two or three times a week, he'd beat her. One time he gave her a black eye, another time he knocked out a tooth. He would tell her she was fat and ugly, and that she should be glad that he wanted to be with her. If she fought back, it was worse. She couldn't call the police because she'd been arrested too many times for sex work and drugs. Sometimes she ran away to the House of the Good Shepherd or the Rainbow House. One time she went to court to file an order of protection, but when she saw Julius at the courthouse, she backed out and said he hadn't done anything. She didn't want to be on the streets, so she stayed. But mostly she stayed because she really loved him.

Laconda felt he really did love her, too, and she needed that love. She was okay with the men coming in, she told me, because she was thinking: It's love. It felt like love because Julius wanted people to see her and be around her and touch her. All her life people called her ugly and nobody wanted her. "I felt beautiful," she said.

In February 2011, Laconda and Julius were at his apartment hanging out and getting ready to do drugs. Laconda wore a long black weave, a black shirt, and black pants. Cocaine was Julius's drug of choice and getting high came with paranoia. That night, the paranoia came fast. He asked Laconda if she was stealing from him and then he said he was going to kill her. She thought he was joking, but then he hit her in the face. She tried to run. First, she headed to the front door, but when he blocked her from leaving, she fled to the kitchen. She was yelling, "I want to go." He was yelling, "Sit your ass down."

He strangled her, and Laconda thought she was going to die, so she grabbed a knife she saw on the kitchen counter and stabbed him in the neck. The blood just poured out of him. Julius's white sweater turned red. There was blood on his blue jeans, briefs, and socks. He died in her arms. She didn't call the police because he was already dead and no one would believe her anyway. He was the only man she had ever loved.

. . .

White-Domain and her team spent five years listening to these women tell their stories, and nothing changed. "It shouldn't take this much work," she told me. "It shouldn't be that we won't send these mothers to prison for more than twenty years only if everything goes right, and if they're lucky enough to get good advocates on their side, and if they're willing to share every ounce of the most horrible things that they are most ashamed of in their lives." White-Domain paused to catch her breath before speaking again. "Because that's what the law asked them to do, and then the law didn't work. Because you can try to explain everything—but it takes too long and it costs too much. It costs too much human effort. The advocacy shouldn't have to be this good. You shouldn't have to try to make judges cry to give Debraca, Angel, and Laconda a shot at getting out of prison to see their kids."

The women were led to believe their stories had power, and they were given the promise of that power, and now what? What else was there? I couldn't think of anything myself.

I had wrongly assumed that if people just understood trauma or if people understood what fear looked like from the women's perspective, they would understand Debraca's response to the landlord's assault. They would understand that she really did believe she was going to die. Same with Angel and Laconda.

"But there's this other piece," White-Domain explained. "What is our tolerance for violence to Black women? Judges and juries wouldn't say they have a high tolerance for violence done to Black women, but that's what the system is telling us. That's the pattern. You know what I mean? That's the racist, patriarchal shit in some people's heads."

I drove back to the airport in silence. I knew now that telling their stories wouldn't change anything for these women, and it was only thinking back to what White-Domain had said that gave me some sense of peace: that one day we might look back and be ashamed about how we treated them.

A couple months later, I called to check in on Laconda. Most days, she woke up at 5:00 a.m., showered, and watched cartoons on PBS until about eight. Then she went to work at the commissary. Usually after work she cried and fell asleep. While Laconda slept, she relived the moment she killed Julius. Night after night, the nightmares rattled her awake, and she cried in the dark. Sometimes she has little daydreams about him too. In the daydreams, they get married and he helps her get her kids back, just like he always promised he would.

No, No, No

I DIDN'T KNOW MUCH ABOUT CHELSEA GODFREY EXCEPT THAT she had gone to trial in 2014 and the man charged with raping her was in prison. I didn't know anything about the case or the accused man. When I reached out to Chelsea, I was working on an article for *The New York Times Magazine* about "freezing," and a retired prosecutor introduced us because she thought Chelsea might have been a survivor who had experienced a frozen response to rape.

I sat down for a video call with Chelsea a few days before Christmas to learn more about her story. I was at a cabin upstate where the owner was convinced his dead wife was sending him messages. While I waited for the call, I kept hearing noises upstairs, and so I was relieved when Chelsea's round, smiling face lit up my screen.

We talked for about an hour and a half, and halfway through our conversation she admitted to me that she had lied in court about how she had responded to the rape as it was happening. She told the court that she had said "no" to him. Now she was telling me she didn't say anything at all.

There's a version of this book in which I withhold this discovery of the woman who lied—a version where I decide not to contaminate the conversation with troubling facts, but this isn't going to be that book because the reason for her lie is an interesting one.

The assault happened on September 7, 2012, during Chelsea's freshman year at Ferrum College in rural southwest Virginia. "There was a guy in my class," she told me, "and he was like, 'Hey, I don't really understand this homework. Do you think you could come help me with it?' And I was like, 'Yeah, well, I'm going to dinner and a movie with my friends, but I'll come over after.' And when I came over, there was no intention of homework. And he was drunk. He assaulted me."

She had looked at the television as it happened. Her only thoughts were, I got to get out of here, I got to get out of here. She told me that she couldn't move until her phone rang and then she could speak and move again. "My roommate is looking for me," Chelsea told him. "She is coming." Her roommate wasn't coming, but she was hoping to scare him. That's when he stopped and he let go of her arm and she rolled to her side.

She remembered him saying: Are you kidding me? I didn't even finish.

While we were talking, she confessed to having lied during her trial, which was at the Franklin County Courthouse in January 2014. Chelsea explained that she had lied in court, not about the rape, but about her response to the rape as it was happening.

"I've always said that I said no," she told me. "But I never did. I never said no, because I couldn't talk. And that's probably the hardest thing, because I have to admit that I lied in court." Chelsea explained that if she hadn't told the court that she said "no," then they wouldn't have believed her. "But I couldn't," Chelsea explained to me. "I was too scared to talk until my phone went off. It was like that fear of if you say no, what's next? So no, I never said no."

I asked if she wanted me to write about her having lied. Because otherwise why would she have admitted this to me? Was this something her lawyers knew about? But she told me she did not want me to mention her confession. She told me to write that she couldn't speak during the rape or that she couldn't remember if she had said "no" or not.

When the call ended, I was alone in the house in the woods again.

I quickly emailed Chelsea, asking her to send me the court transcripts, and while I waited, I wondered about her story. Why would someone admit to lying to a journalist? Especially lying in court? The interview was on the record and intended for a glossy magazine.

And she had already told her story many times at conferences where there were audiences packed with prosecutors and police. She was a speaker with End Violence Against Women International and the Start by Believing program. On the ten-year anniversary of her alleged rape, she told me she was recounting her story when she had a flashback that made her run to the bathroom and cry. The paper trail was long. There was the question of the confession, but also the question of the lie. I was more interested in the question of the lie because it pointed to the fact that she didn't think her response to rape was good enough.

I thought about the fact that it can take time for stories to grow into their fullest forms. If we are scared, or vulnerable, we may discard incomprehensible facts for comprehensible ones. Maybe she had shaped her story to sound like a sensible one? In other words, sometimes we lie to be believed.

Wouldn't it make sense that, if you didn't know that a behavior was normal, you might worry what others would think? That you might disbelieve even yourself?

If she had a name for her behavior, would she have felt the need to lie to be believed? Was she lying to make up for an absence of language?

The lie also made sense in a world that still doesn't want to believe sexual violence is a problem, and where the language to describe ourselves and our fear is insufficient.

But I reread the transcript of our conversation: She told me that her lawyer had told her about "freezing," and that it was normal. Why didn't she offer the truth at that moment?

Sometimes the defenses of our own storytelling can get the best of us.

The author and activist Kalí Tal has written, "Powerful political, economic, and social forces will pressure survivors either to keep their silence or to revise their stories," so that traumatized voices "will be drowned out by those with the influence and resources to silence them, and to trumpet a revised version of their trauma."

If our society expects a certain kind of story, then didn't she give it to us? In the cases of refugees, the best story gets their lives saved. And what counts as best is determined by those in power.

I imagined this same scenario with a friend. If this friend had lied about not fighting back, and then admitted to the lie, I would have thought: That sounds perfectly normal.

But it was different when the lie involved a public accusation or lying in a courtroom under oath.

"But I still didn't consent," Chelsea had told me. "It doesn't make it my fault. I mean, it took me a long time to realize that. But when it first happened, I'm sitting there thinking . . . you couldn't move, you couldn't speak, you didn't say no. So how's anybody going to look at you and think that what happened happened to you? And so I just started telling everyone, 'Well, I said no. I said no.' I was crying. I couldn't move. I think me not moving, me not saying anything, and tears running down my face are clear indications of me saying no without saying no."

After Chelsea reported the rape, the college removed the man from her classes and banned him from her dorm. But she saw him in the cafeteria, lingering around the food. She said he stood with his friends and he pointed and laughed at her.

One day she was in the middle of a quiz when she glanced over at the boy next to her, and he was wearing the same red basketball shorts as the rapist. She sprinted out of the room and thought: I can no longer live this way. She decided to press charges, but when she went to the police, their line of questioning discouraged her again.

She didn't go back to school, but stayed at home in her child-hood bedroom. "I started drinking a lot. I was drinking those really big wine bottles at night. Not the little thin ones. Those big Barefoot ones that are for a whole party. I was the party."

The first time she went to a grand jury her case was rejected. The second time she decided to tell the story herself without a lawyer. This time it worked. The grand jury convened and she got a call from a Commonwealth attorney saying it was a "true bill." She was going to trial. They met in Farmville, Virginia, at the courthouse, to discuss the case. His big find was that she had PCOS and endometriosis, and he learned that sex caused her pain. She spent her senior year of high school in the hospital having back-to-back surgeries. She claimed to have had ten surgeries by the time she went to college. Sex wasn't the first thing on her mind, he argued.

. . .

I received the court transcripts from Chelsea not long after we spoke, and she seemed enthusiastic about my reading them. At the bottom of her email, which was forwarded from her lawyer, he had written: "It's very powerful reading."

The transcript confirmed what she had told me—that she had testified in court to saying "no":

I was asking him to stop and he wouldn't. He was holding my arms and he used his one hand to pull my shorts down. I was crying and I was asking him to stop. I was crying and saying no.

But it was the racial aspects of the case that stood out to me and became central to the story. The accused was a Black man named DaJuan Kirksey.

Q: Did you tell Ms. Legg [an officer] that this would never have happened voluntarily because you would never have sex with a Black man?

A: I didn't say those exact words, but I did say that I would not have sex with a Black man.

I remembered that during our call Chelsea had told me, "They actually tried to tell me, 'Well, do you think maybe it was consensual because he's Black and now you have a problem with it?'" Chelsea added, "They just tried to say that I was a white girl who regretted sleeping with a Black man. And that wasn't, and is not, the case."

A couple months later, I saw the prosecutor who introduced me to Chelsea in Weyers Cave, Virginia, where I was attending a course on trauma and victim behavior for police and prosecutors.

The prosecutor had never represented Chelsea—she only knew about her case because they often traveled the same lecture circuits. "Did you know about this?" I asked, referring to the lie. The prosecutor frowned at the news. "No, no," she said. She shook her head slowly and looked at the ground. She touched her chin and looked back up at me. "No," she said. She asked to read the transcripts. She said she would read them that evening and get back to me the next day.

She was not smiling the next morning. "Can I talk to you for a minute?" she said. We went to a classroom and she closed the door. "I did not sleep," she said. "This is serious."

We tapped pens, drank water, swiveled in our swivel chairs.

This wasn't the news anyone wanted to hear. We spent a few minutes trying to make sense of it. I told the prosecutor my thoughts about storytelling and trauma and how we hadn't named these behaviors for many years. But it was a ridiculous thing to say because the prosecutor was teaching on that very topic.

The prosecutor shook her head. "Maybe Chelsea was lying to you?" she said. She meant lying to me about having lied in court. I had wondered that, too, but it seemed unlikely. "In the end, our theories don't matter," the prosecutor told me, because "the entire trial was based solely on Chelsea's credibility." There was nothing else to go on. There were just two stories, and the jury had chosen to believe Chelsea's story. So now, with this new information, she had lost her credibility.

"We can't sit on this now," the prosecutor said. "I have to send this to my boss. I have to send it to the people around her. I have to get in touch with her therapist." She shook her head and added, "She's very fragile. Her entire identity is a victim."

The prosecutor was right to report what I'd learned, but I wasn't expecting it. I didn't imagine she would take my transcript and distribute it to Chelsea's lawyers. I had only imagined she would talk to Chelsea to figure out what was going on. The prosecutor also told me not to contact her. "It might look like you're tampering with evidence."

What if she really was raped and the lie was just a revision? I didn't want to hurt Chelsea. I didn't want to embarrass her. What if my talking to the prosecutor was doing harm to her? I remembered how she was a mother. I remembered how her child had been sick when we spoke. I remembered how after she was raped Chelsea told me how she had spiraled into self-destruction. That night, I couldn't sleep. My dreams were filled with nightmares. Chelsea was in the dreams, ripping off my face, laughing at me. To report her felt like I was going against everything I had been working toward. When the Innocence Project contacted me a few months later, I had so much anxiety I worried that I was the one in trouble.

I spent hours trying to come to some conclusion about the case until my husband reminded me, "You're not making a decision about the case, you're just telling them what you heard." I was relieved at this thought. In Chelsea's case, as in every case, there is another human being on the other end of the story whose life is shaped by the story she chose to tell. It wasn't just her story, it was a shared story. I thought of DaJuan and his family. A thirty-five-year sentence for a college student in a case without evidence—a case based only on credibility, which was compromised both by her lie and her degrading comments about Black men. If she did lie, as she said she did, she had taken away all the agency of his story.

. . .

I didn't know what to make of a judge who committed a twenty-one-year-old Black student to thirty-five years in prison after Chelsea had conceded at trial that she had told an investigating officer that she "would never have sex with a Black man."

The trial, it just so happens, was in Rocky Mount, Virginia, the seat of Franklin County in the foothills of the Blue Ridge Mountains. Franklin County is nearly 90 percent white and Rocky Mount nearly 70 percent white.

When DaJuan arrived at the courthouse in 2014, he would have passed a statue of a Confederate soldier. A 2020 *Washington Post* article on the county described how a pickup truck accidentally ran into the statue in 2010, and how local officials rebuilt it at a cost of more than $100,000; and "local historians compared its demise to a death in the family." After the Black Lives Matter protests came to town, there was a debate about whether to remove the statue. They left it to the popular vote, and the town voted to leave it. Franklin County is the birthplace of prominent Black educator Booker T. Washington, but the county's historical marker notes only that Confederate "General Jubal A. Early lived in this county." A resident named Jack Eugene Turner was arrested in June 2015 after he hung a Black mannequin by the neck in his front yard to intimidate his Black neighbors.

DaJuan was sentenced to thirty-five years in prison. "If and when you are released," the judge told DaJuan, "then you will be evaluated and most likely declared a sexually violent predator."

———

When the journalist Martenzie Johnson made a list in 2017 for the media platform Andscape of white women who have falsely accused Black men of rape or murder, he wrote: "In each instance the initial story was believable because of the troubling belief that a Black man is capable of such a thing. It's because we've always been told this is what Black men do."

According to the Equal Justice Initiative, a Black person is eight times more likely to be wrongfully convicted than a white person for a crime involving sexual violence. And Black men convicted of raping white women are six times more likely to be innocent than white men convicted of raping white women.

Scholars have written that the sexualization of Black men in America began during slavery: when Black men were forced to rape female slaves for the purpose of creating more slaves, when Black men were punished with sexual assault, and when Black men were victims of sexual violence perpetrated by white women on plantations. However, the "most virulent racist ideology about Black male sexuality," writes Martha Hodes in *White Women, Black Men: Illicit Sex in the South,* "emerged in the decades that followed the Civil War." During Reconstruction, white men were threatened by newly freed Black men, and racial tensions were "expressed in sexual terms" to sideline the question of race. Black men having sex with white women was, as Hodes put it, "a new language of sexualized politics."

I had visited the women's prison around the time the Innocence Project took on DaJuan's case. Their stories haunted this one. The words of Rachel White-Domain kept coming back to me: how the foundation of sexual-assault laws in America were based on a fantasy that white women needed protection from being raped by Black men. How Black men were lynched and burned alive for false accusations of rape. "And so, historically, we have always deferred to the white woman," White-Domain told me. "And the Black man has been the accused."

As Paula Giddings, a professor at Smith College, has pointed out in her writing on race and sexuality, while Black men are being falsely accused of rape, Black women are actually being raped.

Almost a year after I talked to the prosecutor, lawyers investigating the case at the Innocence Project called to tell me that they found "no evidence of rape."

The case was relitigated in March 2024, and Chelsea was charged with "fraud against the court." DaJuan's family was in attendance. I was going to be called as a witness, but my deposition and the transcripts were enough.

I thought DaJuan should be released. We have always given white women the benefit of the doubt. Why not give it to DaJuan?

"They asked me to pass along their thanks to you," one of the caseworkers told me on behalf of DaJuan's family. "No matter what happens, they are very grateful that when you thought something was wrong with this case, you took it to the appropriate person in a position to handle it and notify the prosecutor. They asked me to pass along their gratitude." But even after Chelsea admitted to giving a jury false information, nothing changed. DaJuan is still in prison.

I kept coming back to the words of Jean McAllister, a social worker who has served as an expert on sexual-assault cases for over forty years. "We think we know these stories," she told me, "because we hear about them in the news, because of the Weinstein trial and maybe the Cosby trial, all these celebrity cases. But otherwise, we don't really hear these everyday stories. We don't know anything."

Luisa's Escape

LUISA SCHNEIDER DIDN'T WANT TO TALK TO DARREN, SO SHE escaped to her bedroom. He followed. "What did he do to you?" he asked. And when Luisa didn't reply, he said, "Did he rape you?" Darren took her hand, and she pulled it away.

"Please," he said, and he took her hand again.

He moved his index finger up her wrist and forearm, and her entire body shook. It felt as if she were with the man again, with his hands on her spine, unable to breathe.

Luisa lived with Darren and eight others in a yellow house along a dirt road in the hillside community of Allentown, in eastern Freetown, Sierra Leone, where she had lived for the last five years.

She told Darren she didn't want anyone to know what had happened to her. It was a way of denying the reality of what she had experienced.

Luisa was a doctoral student at Oxford, doing anthropological fieldwork on Ebola survivors. It was the summer of 2017, and the man who did it, the one who raped her, was the head of the group she was studying—the gatekeeper of her research.

Luisa recounted this scene when she wrote about the rape and its aftermath in the anthropology journal *Ethos*. "My world felt sterile, cold, without sound, color, or smell," she wrote.

"And I was under." Luisa thought she was acting normal—the way she had seen sexually assaulted women act in Western movies: as if she had wiggled into a crack in the wall and was looking out at the world.

But Darren, who is from Sierra Leone, was panicking about Luisa's passive response. He worried that the rapist had left something—his energy and his power—inside her and that the bond between them would grow until she went to a medicine man who had the power to wash the residue of the rapist from her body.

Mohammed, her research assistant, told Luisa that he believed the same thing: that the rapist would control her through his semen. A medicine man needed to destroy this bond. If she didn't do it quickly, the rapist would have power over her, and the bond would grow stronger until it would be impossible to break.

"He will forever be connected to you," Darren had told Luisa.

Luisa said it all didn't matter, because she had been violently raped and the harm was done. Darren told her no—the harm had just begun.

Luisa did not want to listen to these men talk about a connection between her and her rapist, and she didn't want to go to a medicine man who would make her get naked and drink a bad-tasting drink to extinguish this mysterious bond with the rapist. "I did not want to elevate his power by considering his semen to have uncanny qualities," Luisa wrote in *Ethos*.

Instead, she bathed herself over and over to rid herself of any residue of the man and his semen.

She didn't want to tell anyone what happened, but soon she had to tell her supervisors so they would know why she stopped doing research for her PhD. She also told a few friends, her partner, and her mother, and then she put the memory away. "I then began compartmentalizing the rape as an incident that I could isolate and separate from life and people," she wrote, "stuff into a locked box in the most remote corner of my consciousness to starve it of all attention until it died."

The next four years, she told me, were haunted ones. A panther stalked her dreams. An invisible hand grabbed at her back. When she looked at her own hands, she saw the rapist holding them. He visited her while she slept, stared at her through tram windows. The faces of men who came close to her face morphed into his.

The rapist lived through her body, existing and experiencing every part of her life alongside her. She seemed to always feel his hand on her back, moving up her spine. It left her shaking. She swapped her double mattress for a twin that she pushed against the wall. She made herself small and never asked for help because she didn't want to be a burden. She stayed quiet and never repeated herself. She stopped exercising and stopped eating well. She imagined herself to be ruined and undeserving of love and so she refused love whenever it was offered. She didn't touch herself and didn't let others touch her either. Sex was an out-of-body experience and she puposefully suffocated all desire.

She kept thinking: It will get better, it will go away. And it never did. When she looked at her naked body, she felt disgust.

When she returned to Europe, it seemed as if everyone assumed the violence had changed her for the worse, but they also assumed she would get over it. They thought one day she would be her old self again. And her European friends would always make sure to try to tell her that she was "okay." She remembered a friend saying, I've been watching you and you seem "okay." You're fine now, everything's fine. Luisa heard it so often that she started telling herself that she was in fact "okay." It was a big responsibility to always have to be "okay," especially because sometimes she didn't feel that way: There were still hands on her spine and the panther in her dreams.

She had to do something to get better, and she started reading European self-help blogs and forums about "surviving rape." They all said things like Center yourself, or Become a strong survivor. They made healing all about putting yourself back together, because you have been "shattered" and "ruined" by rape. "Healing," according to everything she read, meant going back into the world exactly as she had been before the rape.

But she couldn't seem to get back to the way she had been. On good days, when she went out and did things without fear, she felt like a success. On bad days, when she trembled or couldn't socialize, she felt like a failure. Everything was about binaries.

Friends seemed disappointed in this fact—that she was not the same as she had once been. It was tiring. The expectations of "resilience" made her feel like she was constantly failing. No one wanted to hang out with a sad woman who was trapped in the past. They wanted her story to look different from the reality of what she was experiencing. She was not okay. She did not feel like a "survivor."

As the blogs recommended, she also tried saying "my rape," to give herself ownership over the event and its consequences. It was a way of speaking about violence that many Westerners used to describe rape. *My* rape or *my* assault.

———

Seven years passed and Luisa still wasn't doing okay. She could not erase the violence. She could not become someone who lived as if it hadn't happened. There was no resurrection. How wrong she had been about stuffing the memory into a box with the hope that it would wither and die.

But she did notice something interesting—how different the responses were among her friends in Sierra Leone compared with her friends in Europe.

Back in Sierra Leone, she had waited seven months before she told her housemates what had happened to her. "No one in Sierra Leone was surprised," she told me over the phone. In fact, "they already knew because they could see it on me." The way Darren had also been able to "see it on her." No one saw her differently because of the rape, and no one made a big deal of it either. They didn't ask her any questions, but simply shared their own experiences of suffering and violence.

One woman shared that her parents had given her away and that she grew up with her aunt, but that her aunt didn't want her either, so she was passed along to someone else. Another said she hid from soldiers during the war, unsure if she would be found. Another talked about her own experience of sexual violence.

They didn't ask anything more about Luisa's experience.

She thought this was strange, but was also relieved she didn't have to talk more about what happened to her.

As the years passed, she realized that she had in fact been living "the bond" that Darren and Mohammed warned her about. She was living it in the form of flashbacks, distortions, and nightmares. "It really felt as if I were living with a controlling partner," she told me. Darren and Luisa had been using different terminologies, but they were describing the same thing. And while Darren wanted her to use coping mechanisms that involved the community, Luisa had wanted to carry the burden alone.

Unlike the individualistic culture of Germany, where Luisa was raised, or the United Kingdom, where she did her PhD, Sierra Leone was a collective culture, which meant you were still your own person, with your own dreams and goals, but these were always in relation to other people. A personally experienced trauma was expected to be felt by family and community, and no one was expected to suffer alone. The self was relational and fluid. Pain was not held by a single person, which would make it heavy and a burden, but by everyone, which stole pain's power and diluted it. The anthropologist Arthur Kirmayer has written that in collectivist cultures "the notion of personhood does not coincide with the boundary of the skin." An individual was defined through the family and the community. If you were already part of a community, then you couldn't be completely ruined by an experience.

"What happens then is you take care of each other in a different way," Luisa told me. "If somebody else is unwell, then the entire community becomes sick. You suffer from somebody else suffering. Your well-being is inside you, but it is also all around you." She explained that so much of therapy in the Western world is about boundary work and about understanding that someone else's problem isn't your problem. "But in a collective community," she said, "you would say, for example, 'Well, of course you're not well, your mother isn't well, so let's try to make her well.'"

Luisa was beginning to understand that she was responding to sexual violence with European and American cultural scripts, and that all these beliefs were part of a Western way of thinking about and expressing trauma. For Luisa, they weren't working to help her heal or make sense of what happened.

While Luisa had seen the rape as a defining moment that

had shattered a previously intact being, her Sierra Leonean friends saw wounds as integral to their sense of self. While they saw the rape as the beginning of a relationship with her rapist, she saw it as the end of her relationship with herself as a person who was okay. While Darren and Mohammed saw coping as a survival strategy rooted in the community, Luisa believed she had to cope alone. She began to understand that the Western way of thinking was more about banishing and erasing the experience of rape, which also meant overcoming it in a linear way. Her Sierra Leonean friends saw continuity in time, whereas Luisa saw the event as a rupture in time that had turned her life into a before and an after. While Luisa felt the trauma in her body, she had thought only "thinking through" and "speaking about" what happened to her could offer her peace.

Luisa told me how she started reading books on postcolonial trauma narratives, questioning how Western ideas of trauma had shaped her response: How it meant coping alone, ignoring the body, trying to live as if the rape hadn't happened at all. How uncertainty in Western culture was thought of as a problem, while safety and stability were considered normal, so that when something tragic happened, it was all about rebuilding the groundwork to get things back to the way they were before. "But it's actually strange," Luisa said, "because lives are so much more complicated than safety as default or stability as default." Her Sierra Leonean friends saw wounds, illness, breakups, suffering, and violence as integral to their sense of self. That it was impossible for her not to be okay, even temporarily, was a Western way of looking at trauma.

· · ·

Luisa didn't think these revelations meant completely giving up her old beliefs or that a medicine man would have cured her. Not at all. But it was helpful to question her own beliefs about what trauma, and our responses to it, should look like.

"The way forward is not just to go all in," she told me. "If we're decolonizing, we're not recentering something else, we are just allowing multiplicity to be."

Luisa realized that calling the violence "my rape" stopped her from seeing that the violence was also a social issue, which helped her see her rapist not just as someone who made the choice to harm her, but also as a product of systems and structures. "There's a danger of suffering alone," she realized.

And the more she read about the Western hegemony on trauma, the less often she saw the panther in her dreams.

When a friend learned Luisa was still struggling to look at herself—at her naked body—without disgust, she recommended Luisa "explore her body with her own hands—see how it feels, see how nice it is."

Which body? Luisa wondered. She had already "discarded [her] body." It belonged only to him.

For years she couldn't see her body through her own eyes, only the eyes of the rapist. It was like she had floated up into his gaze and stayed trapped in his eyes.

Luisa's friend told her that once she had new memories, then she should look at herself again. If she still couldn't look at her naked body, then she should start by closing her eyes.

That's how Luisa began: feeling her body with her eyes closed, slowly, letting her hands gain perspective and sight. She tried to create new ways of seeing her body, starting with what her friends in Sierra Leone saw when they looked at her. She realized that other people didn't see the body she saw, and that what she saw on her body was a memory, not an ongoing experience.

When she returned to Sierra Leone to start research on a new dissertation, she practiced seeing herself through the eyes of the community. They didn't see the hands moving up her spine. They didn't see a raped body, they saw Luisa. They recognized the pain, but it wasn't what defined her.

In Luisa's ethnography *Love and Violence in Sierra Leone: Mediating Intimacy After Conflict,* she recalled an elder saying: "You stayed here after the rape. We saw you suffer, so we trust you to understand our own suffering."

They saw her as an academic with a notebook and a new project on love and violence in Sierra Leone.

These were new memories she gained from looking through the eyes of others.

When she was ready, she tried to see herself again with her own eyes.

She sees herself on Naimbana Street, with the smells of spiced beef, chicken on grills, banana fritters, steamed fish. There are plantains, yams, cassava, the undertones of tropical fruit.

She sees herself standing on the veranda of the house she shares with Darren and Mohammed, looking out at Tagrin Bay, out at the swamps.

She sees herself listening to the ordinary dreams and desires, pains and failures, of hundreds of people in the community while working on her new dissertation about love and violence in Sierra Leone. She sees that she is someone who is no longer asked to leave during domestic disputes because she is now someone they can trust. She sees herself in overwhelmed pain when she listens to these fights, but she tries to share this pain with as many people as she can. She remembers trying not to be alone.

She remembers early mornings under the mango tree with girls from the beauty salon, braiding hair, sharing gossip.

She sees that her body lives among the community, responding to these new memories and sensations, unlike before, when she felt nothing and there was only a single memory that pulled her away from the present and back into the arms of the rapist.

Soon she came out of the crack in the wall, out of the black hole. Sounds returned with an enormous whack. The bread was eaten. The smoke of cassava was inhaled with a choke. Finally her feet touched the floor, finally felt the earth. Her body surfaced with force.

She began to see herself again. She forgot all about telling her story, speaking her story. She just kept looking at her body, discarding the rapist's gaze.

And that was how she escaped him.

Down Below

THERE IS A DARK SIDE TO SELF-PRESERVATION. OUR DEFENSES keep us safe but draw us into their imprisoning powers. We go under. Sometimes it looks like paralysis, psychic retreats, unconscious sanctuaries, utopian escapes.

When Luisa Schneider fell to the ground, pushed by the man's hands, she fell to the floor, but she did not stop there. "I drifted below its visible materiality to a place that had now become my world," she wrote. "And I was under."

At the start of the war, after her husband was taken, after dead bodies piled up, and after she was raped, the surrealist writer and painter Leonora Carrington went "down below." In her memoir by the same name, she writes about the sensation of being pulled toward the ground until her face was flat on it and she "was being completely absorbed by the earth," and how, suddenly, she walked with "tremendous effort in some matter as thick as mud."

Soon after, when Carrington was institutionalized at a mental hospital in Spain, a nurse asked, "Where do you come from?" And Carrington responded, "From down below."

Persephone went down below after she was abducted and raped by Hades. She lived half her life belowground among the dead, and half above among the living, cycling in and out of the underworld between seasons. She became a woman who lived in both worlds; as if survival meant being born again and again, and a visit to the underworld of trauma was an essential part of a woman's experience. But sometimes we get lost in our own survival strategies. We stay down below.

My husband and I went out to dinner the other day, to a sushi restaurant. We were waiting outside and there were people around us waiting too. We were chatting with each other among the people, sharing stories, looking at the menu, checking the weather. He had just told a story, I don't remember what it was about, but I could not really listen and I could not respond. Nearby I saw a man: a green shirt, a damp shirt.

A man coming near, standing too close. He left me wordless and staring.

"What's wrong?" my husband said.

I felt the shadow of something moving overhead, a quiet flapping, my body rising.

I was down below. It was just for a moment, suspended. A woman mesmerized. I heard the hymn in the violence. And then, seconds later, I was back. My husband put his arms around me. He was used to it by now. "Was it the man?" he said.

A few years ago, in Oregon, I met a teen girl in a loose lavender hoodie and low bootcut jeans. We looked at each other across the generations, across desert and forest, her blue eyes narrowing. We were at the fairgrounds on muddy ground coated with bits of hay. Everywhere around us were kids with animals. They were showing the animals at the fair. This girl was very small, but beside her was an enormous bull. He was matted in places with the coloring of maple syrup. The horns curved before going erect. Green flies glittered around his eyes.

The bull had been causing trouble. "An intense creature," she said. Earlier he nearly trampled a toddler. Grown men flung themselves on the bull, but the animal kicked them. This girl told me that she walked up to the bull and put a ring in his nose. It calmed him right down. "People say it's inhumane," she told me. "But it just pinches. That's all."

Now she was a one-hundred-pound kid leading this bull around. I saw myself in the girl. I recognized her terror and the fascination of the bull.

"Some people only know about the bull from a distance," she explained. "But have they ever held that much power in their hands? Do they really know what it means to lead that much power?"

She held out the rope to me. She thought she had stopped the violence of the bull. She wanted to share this with me by explaining her power, and letting me feel what it was like to have that power. Was it the same power the predator has to freeze prey?

Who holds who? I could not tell.

All I could see was that she was still tied to the bull, and when she let go, that power was gone.

Acknowledgments

Thomas Gebremedhin, friend and brilliant editor, who believed in this book and stuck with me to the end. Thank you for your insight, for your fearlessness to push against convention, and for being someone who can truly pull a writer out of the woods and into the light.

Jin Auh, my incredible agent, whose enthusiasm and faith in this book helped make it a reality, even at its messiest, weirdest, and most unformed stage.

The tremendous team at Doubleday, for bringing this book into the world, especially Johanna Zwirner, Elena Hershey, Anne Jaconette, Anna Carson, and Jane Cavolina.

Sarah Jean Grimm and Whitney Peeling at Broadside: I adore you both and I'm so grateful for the energy you put into this book.

Oliver Munday for the perfect cover.

Claire Gutierrez and everyone at *The New York Times Magazine* who published my work over the years, especially Jessica Lustig, Bill Wasik, Jake Silverstein, Jane Ackerman, and Steven Stern.

The literary journals where snippets of memoir originally appeared: the *Indiana Review*, the *Literary Review*, the *American Literary Review*.

Alex Mar, Bee Sacks, Adrienne Raphel, Helen Rubenstein, and Dina Nayeri for being stellar readers. Tony Tulathimutte for all the anecdotes about freezing. Rayan El-Amine for being an incred-

Acknowledgments

ible research assistant. David Morris for the conversation about trauma and women's storytelling. Tommy Wisdom for connecting me to one of my subjects. The journalism department at New York University, especially Rob Boyton and Ted Conover. And all my students for inspiring me.

Tom Colligan for fact-checking these pages and making the book so much better.

All the survivors, experts, activists, organizers, fighters who spoke to me. Thank you for your words and stories. There would be no book without you.

My mother and father for all their support and for bringing me into the wilds to learn about the animals and the trees. My brother Ben, his wife Lisa, and his kids, Madeline and Connor, for always cheering me on. Baby Ilya who was born in the middle of writing this book: You bring me so much joy. And everyone who helped with childcare: Yin, Carola, Jane, Rosa, Sarah. And Donna, for hours of laughter at "the beach."

Finally, my husband Alexander, this book would not exist without you. Your love buoyed me through this book. Thank you for letting me go into the underworld and for welcoming me back with open arms upon my return. I love you.

Bibliography

Girl in the Snow

Duras, Marguerite. *The Lover.* Translated by Barbara Bray. New York: Pantheon, 1985.

Garner, Helen. *The First Stone: Some Difficult Questions About Sex and Power.* Sydney: Picador/Pan Macmillan Australia, 1995.

Oates, Joyce Carol. "The Knife." In *Heat and Other Stories.* New York: Dutton, 1991.

Thompson, Zoë Brigley. "Beyond Symbolic Rape: The Insidious Trauma of Conquest in Marguerite Duras's *The Lover* and Eileen Chang's 'Lust, Caution.'" *Feminist Formations* 28, no. 3 (2016): 1–26.

Bewilderment

Maynard, Nettie Colburn. *Was Abraham Lincoln a Spiritualist?* Philadelphia: R. C. Hartranft, 1891.

Moore, Laurence. "The Spiritualist Medium: A Study of Female Professionalism in Victorian America." *American Quarterly* 27, no. 2 (1975).

Prophet, Erin. *Prophet's Daughter: My Life with Elizabeth Clare Prophet Inside the Church Universal and Triumphant.* Self-published, 2010.

Whitsel, Bradley C. *The Church Universal and Triumphant: Elizabeth Clare Prophet's Apocalyptic Movement.* New York: Syracuse University Press, 2003.

Bibliography

What I Look Like When I'm Afraid

Bankey, Ruth. "La Donna é Mobile: Constructing the Irrational Woman." *Gender, Place & Culture: A Journal of Feminist Geography* 8, no. 1 (2001): 37–54.

———. Review of *The Agoraphobic Condition*, by Paul Carter and Joyce Davidson. *Cultural Geographies* 11, no. 3 (2004): 347–55.

Davidson, Joyce. "Fear and Trembling in the Mall: Women, Agoraphobia and Body Boundaries." In *Geographies of Women's Health*, edited by I. Dyck, N. Davis Lewis, and S. McLafferty, 213–30. London: Routledge, 2001.

———. " '. . . The World Was Getting Smaller': Women, Agoraphobia and Bodily Boundaries." *Area* 32 (2005): 31–40.

Deutsch, Helene. "The Genesis of Agoraphobia." *International Journal of Psychoanalysis* 10 (1929): 51–69.

Elmazzahi, Dina, and Jihad Abuseif. "The Era of Agoraphobia: Evaluation of the Public Spaces in Alexandria." *Trialog* 4 (2020): 18–24.

Elsenga, Simon, and Paul M. G. Emmelkamp. "Behavioral Treatment of an Incest-Related Trauma in an Agoraphobic Client." *Journal of Anxiety Disorders* 4, no. 2 (1990): 151–62.

Gelfond, Marjorie. "Reconceptualizing Agoraphobia: A Case Study of Epistemological Bias in Clinical Research." *Feminism and Psychology* 1, no. 2 (1991): 247–62.

Graham, Caveney. *On Agoraphobia*. London: Picador, 2023.

Hafner, R. J. "Predicting the Effects on Husbands of Behaviour Therapy for Wives' Agoraphobia." *Behaviour Research and Therapy* 22, no. 3 (1984): 217–26.

Hoagwood, Kimberly. "Poststructuralist Historicism and the Psychological Construction of Anxiety Disorders." *Journal of Psychology* 127, no. 1 (1993): 105–22.

Holmes, Joshua. "Space and the Secure Base in Agoraphobia: A Qualitative Survey." *Area* 40, no. 3 (2008): 375–82.

Keire, Mara. "Shouting Abuse, Harmless Jolly, and Promiscuous Flattery: Considering the Contours of Sexual Harassment at Macy's Department Store, 1910–1915." *Labor: Studies in Working-Class History* 19, no. 1 (2022): 52–73.

Knapp, Terry J. *Westphal's "Die Agoraphobie" with Commentary: The*

Bibliography

Beginnings of Agoraphobia. Translated by Michael T. Schumacher. Millburn, NJ: University Press of America, 1988.

Kuch, K., and R. P. Swinson. "Agoraphobia: What Westphal Really Said." *Canadian Journal of Psychiatry. Revue Canadienne de Psychiatrie* 37, no. 2 (1992): 133–36.

Loper, A. B., and N. Kassam-Adams. "Anxiety Disorders in Women." *IRIS: A Journal About Women* 31 (1994): 28–34.

Mairs, Nancy. *Carnal Acts.* Boston: Beacon Press, 1996.

———. *Plaintext.* Tucson: University of Arizona Press, 1986.

McHugh, Maureen C. "A Feminist Approach to Agoraphobia: Challenging Traditional Views of Women at Home." In *Lectures on the Psychology of Women*, 4th ed., edited by Joan C. Chrisler, Carla Golden, and Patricia D. Rozee, 393–417. New York: McGraw-Hill, 2008.

McTeague, Lisa M., et al. "Aversive Imagery in Panic Disorder: Agoraphobia Severity, Comorbidity, and Defensive Physiology." *Biological Psychiatry* 70, no. 5 (2011): 415–24.

Reuter, Shelley Zipora. "'The Very Opposite of Calm': A Socio-Cultural History of Agoraphobia." PhD diss., Queen's University, 2001.

Seidenberg, Robert, and Karen DeCrow. *Women Who Marry Houses: Panic and Protest in Agoraphobia.* New York: McGraw-Hill, 1983.

Siegel, Suzie. "Safe at Home: Agoraphobia and the Discourse on Women's Place." PhD diss., University of South Florida, 2001.

Spineanu, Eugenia. *Agoraphobia Unveiled.* Independently published, 2024.

Sutherland, Henry. "On 'Agoraphobia.'" *Journal of Psychological Medicine and Mental Pathology* 3, no. 2 (1877): 265–69.

Trotter, David. "The Invention of Agoraphobia." *Victorian Literature and Culture* 32, no. 2 (2004): 463–74.

Vidler, Anthony. *Warped Space: Art, Architecture, and Anxiety in Modern Culture.* Cambridge, MA: MIT Press, 2000.

Walkowitz, Judith R. "Going Public: Shopping, Street Harassment, and Streetwalking in Late Victorian London." *Representations* 62 (1998): 1–30.

Werner, W. L. "The Psychology of Marcel Proust." *The Sewanee Review* 39, no. 3 (1931): 276–81.

Bibliography

Yates, Sheena. "Agoraphobia and Melancholia: Thoughts on Milrod's 'Emptiness in Agoraphobia Patients.'" *Journal of the American Psychoanalytic Association* 63, no. 4 (2015): 695–725.

Yonkers, Kimberly A. "Panic and Agoraphobia: Gender as a Factor." *CNS Spectrums* 9, no. 9 (2004): 6–7.

The Frozen Ones

Abrams, Murray P., R. Nicholas Carleton, Steven Taylor, and Gordon J. G. Asmundson. "Human Tonic Immobility: Measurement and Correlates." *Depression and Anxiety* 26 (2009): 550–56.

Arnsten, Amy F. T. "Stress Weakens Prefrontal Networks: Molecular Insults to Higher Cognition." *Nature Neuroscience* 18, no. 10 (October 2015): 1376–84.

Baines, Barbara J. "Effacing Rape in Early Modern Representation." *ELH* 65, no. 1 (Spring 1998): 69–98.

Basile, Giambattista. "Sun, Moon, and Talia." Italy: 1634.

Bourke, Joanna. "A Global History of Sexual Violence." Lecture, November 22, 2017.

———. *Rape: A Cultural History from 1860 to the Present.* New York: Shoemaker and Hoard, 2007.

———. *Rape: Sex, Violence, History.* Berkeley, CA: Counterpoint Press, 2007.

———. "Sexual Violence, Bodily Pain, and Trauma: A History." *Theory, Culture & Society* 29, no. 3 (2012): 25–31.

Bovin, Michelle J., Shari Jager-Hyman, Sari D. Gold, Brian P. Marx, and Denise M. Sloan. "Tonic Immobility Mediates the Influence of Peritraumatic Fear and Perceived Inescapability on Posttraumatic Stress Symptom Severity Among Sexual Assault Survivors." *Journal of Traumatic Stress* 21, no. 4 (August 2008): 402–9.

Bracha, H. Stefan. "Freeze, Flight, Fight, Fright, Faint: Adaptationist Perspectives on the Acute Stress Response Spectrum." *CNS Spectrums* 9, no. 9 (September 2004): 679–85.

Brown, Laura S. "Not Outside the Range: One Feminist Perspective on Psychic Trauma." In *Trauma: Explorations in Memory*, edited by Cathy Caruth, 100–12. Baltimore: Johns Hopkins University Press, 1995.

Burgess, Ann Wolbert, and Lynda Lytle Holmstrom. "Coping Behavior of the Rape Victim." *American Journal of Psychiatry* 133, no. 4 (April 1976): 413–18.

———. "Rape Trauma Syndrome." *American Journal of Psychiatry* 131, no. 9 (September 1974): 981–86.

Burr, Viv, and Jeff Hearn, eds. *Sex, Violence and the Body: The Erotics of Wounding.* London: Palgrave Macmillan, 2008.

Campbell, Kirsten. "Legal Memories: Sexual Assault Memory and International Humanitarian Law." *Signs: Journal of Women in Culture and Society* 28, no. 1 (2002): 149–78.

Cannon, W. B. *Bodily Changes in Pain, Hunger, Fear and Rage: An Account of Recent Researches.* London: Kegan Paul, 1915.

Caruth, Cathy. *Unclaimed Experience: Trauma, Narrative, and History.* Baltimore: Johns Hopkins University Press, 1996.

———, ed. *Testimony: Crises of Witnessing in Literature, Psychoanalysis, and History.* New York: Routledge, 1992.

Connell, Patricia. "Understanding Victimization and Agency: Considerations of Race, Class, and Gender." *PoLAR* 20, no. 2 (1997): 115–43.

Darnton, Robert. *Mesmerism and the End of the Enlightenment in France.* Cambridge, MA: Harvard University Press, 1968.

de Heer, Brooke A., and Lynn C. Jones. "Investigating the Self-Protective Potential of Immobility in Victims of Rape." *Violence and Victims* 32, no. 2 (2017): 210–19.

Duddle, M. "Emotional Sequelae of Sexual Assault." *Journal of the Royal Society of Medicine* 84, no. 1 (1991): 26–28.

Dunn, Caroline. "The Language of Ravishment in Medieval England." *Speculum* 86, no. 1 (January 2011): 79–116.

Elliott, Audrea E., and Mark G. Packard. "Intra-Amygdala Anxiogenic Drug Infusion Prior to Retrieval Biases Rats Towards the Use of Habit Memory." *Neurobiology of Learning and Memory* 90 (2008): 616–23.

Ellison, Louise, and Vanessa E. Munro. "Reacting to Rape: Exploring Mock Jurors' Assessments of Complainant Credibility." *British Journal of Criminology* 48 (2009): 1–18.

———. "Turning Mirrors into Windows? Assessing the Impact of (Mock) Juror Education in Rape Trials." *British Journal of Criminology* 49 (2009): 363–83.

Even, Yael. "Daphne (Without Apollo) Reconsidered: Some Disregarded Images of Sexual Pursuit in Italian Renaissance and Baroque Art." *Studies in Iconography* 18 (1997): 143–59.

Ferguson, Frances. "Rape and the Rise of the Novel." *Representations* 20 (Autumn 1987): 88–112.

Fisher, H. E., L. L. Brown, A. Aron, G. Strong, and D. Mashek. "Reward, Addiction, and Emotion Regulation Systems Associated with Rejection in Love." *Journal of Neurophysiology* 104, no. 1 (2010): 51–60.

Fusé, Tiffany, John P. Forsyth, Brian Marx, Gordon G. Gallup, and Scott Weaver. "Factor Structure of the Tonic Immobility Scale in Female Sexual Assault Survivors: An Exploratory and Confirmatory Factor Analysis." *Journal of Anxiety Disorders* 21 (2007): 265–83.

Gallup, Gordon G., Jr. "Animal Hypnosis: Factual Status of a Fictional Concept." *Psychological Bulletin* 81, no. 11 (1974): 836–53.

Gasbarri, Antonella, Assunta Pompili, Mark G. Packard, and Carlos Tomaz. "Habit Learning and Memory in Mammals: Behavioral and Neural Characteristics." *Neurobiology of Learning and Memory* 114 (2014): 198–208.

Geraerts, Elke, Harald Merckelbach, Marko Jelicic, Elke Smeets, and Jaap van Heerden. "Dissociative Symptoms and How They Relate to Fantasy Proneness in Women Reporting Repressed or Recovered Memories." *Personality and Individual Differences* 40 (2006): 1143–51.

Gilbert, Paula. *Violence and the Female Imagination: Quebec's Women Writers Re-Frame Gender in North American Cultures*. Montreal: McGill-Queen's University Press, 2006.

Gutmann, Matthew. "The Animal Inside: Men and Violence." *Current Anthropology* 62 (2020): 183–92.

Harsey, Sarah J., and Jennifer J. Freyd. "Defamation and DARVO." *Journal of Trauma & Dissociation* 23, no. 5 (2022): 1–9.

Harsey, Sarah J., Eileen L. Zurbriggen, and Jennifer J. Freyd. "Perpetrator Responses to Victim Confrontation: DARVO and Victim Self-Blame." *Journal of Aggression, Maltreatment & Trauma* 26, no. 6 (2017): 644–63.

Hawksley, Lucinda. *Lizzie Siddal: The Tragedy of a Pre-Raphaelite Supermodel*. London: Andre Deutsch, 2004.

Henning, Kris, Angela R. Jones, and Robert Holdford. " 'I Didn't Do

It, but If I Did I Had a Good Reason": Minimization, Denial, and Attributions of Blame Among Male and Female Domestic Violence Offenders." *Journal of Family Violence* 20, no. 3 (June 2005): 131–39.

Humphreys, Kathryn L., Colin L. Sauder, Elaine K. Martin, and Brian P. Marx. "Tonic Immobility in Childhood Sexual Abuse Survivors and Its Relationship to Posttraumatic Stress Symptomatology." *Journal of Interpersonal Violence* 25, no. 2 (February 2010): 358–73.

Jaekl, Phil. *Out Cold: A Chilling Descent in the Macabre Controversial Lifesaving History of Hypothermia.* New York: PublicAffairs, 2021.

Kinports, Kit. "Rape and Force: The Forgotten Mens Rea." *Buffalo Criminal Law Review* 4, no. 2 (January 2001): 755–99.

Kozlowska K., P. Walker, L. McLean, and P. Carrive. "Fear and the Defense Cascade: Clinical Implications and Management." *Harvard Review of Psychiatry* 23, no. 4 (2015): 263–87.

Lauderdale, Helen J. "The Admissibility of Expert Testimony on Rape Trauma Syndrome." *Journal of Criminal Law and Criminology* 75, no. 4 (Winter 1984): 1366–1416.

Luckhurst, Roger. "The Science-Fictionalization of Trauma: Remarks on Narratives of Alien Abduction." *Science Fiction Studies* 25, no. 1 (March 1998): 29–52.

Maddaus, Gene. "Read Jessica Mann's Full Victim-Impact Statement from the Harvey Weinstein Sentencing." *Variety*, March 11, 2020.

Michaels, Paula A., and Christina Twomey. *Gender and Trauma Since 1900.* London: Bloomsbury, 2021.

Moskowitz, Andrew. "Dissociation and Violence: A Review of the Literature." *Trauma, Violence & Abuse* 5, no. 1 (January 2004): 21–46.

Ovid. *Metamorphoses.* Translated by Rolfe Humphries. Bloomington: Indiana University Press, 1960.

Pernoud, Hermeline. "Fantasizing *The Sleeping Beauty*: Rape Culture and Consent in Contemporary Reminiscences of a Fairy Tale." *Sociopoétiques* 4 (2019).

Sweet, John Wood. *The Sewing Girl's Tale: A Story of Crime and Consequences in Revolutionary America.* New York: Henry Holt & Co., 2022.

Tsur, Noga, and Carmit Katz. " 'And Then Cinderella Was Lying in My Bed': Dissociation Displays in Forensic Interviews with Children Following Intrafamilial Child Sexual Abuse." *Journal of Interpersonal Violence* 37, no. 17–18 (2021).

Zweig, Stefan. *Mental Healers.* Translated by Eden and Cedar Paul. New York: Viking Press, 1932.

Rapture

Adams, Carol J., and Josephine Donovan, eds. *Animals & Women: Feminist Theoretical Explorations.* Durham, NC: Duke University Press, 1995.

Arva, Eugene L. *The Traumatic Imagination: Histories of Violence in Magical Realist Fiction.* Amherst, NY: Cambria Press, 2011.

Birke, Lynda. *Feminism, Animals, and Science: The Naming of the Shrew.* Philadelphia: Open University Press, 1994.

Campbell, Bradley A., Rachel K. Carter, David S. Lapsey Jr., and R. Edward Carter. "An Evaluation of Victim Centered, Trauma Informed Interview Training for Sexual Assault Investigators Using Standardized Patient Actors: A Randomized Controlled Trial: Kentucky, 2019–2022." Final research report, University of Louisville, June 30, 2022.

Chesler, Phyllis. *Women and Madness.* New York: Palgrave Macmillan, 2005.

Cvetkovich, Ann. *An Archive of Feeling: Trauma, Sexuality, and Lesbian Public Cultures.* Durham, NC: Duke University Press, 2003.

Gravdal, Kathryn. *Ravishing Maidens: Writing Rape in Medieval French Literature and Law.* Philadelphia: University of Pennsylvania Press, 1991.

Gravlee, Clarence C. "How Race Becomes Biology: Embodiment of Social Inequality." *American Journal of Physical Anthropology* 139, no. 1 (2009): 47–57.

Haaken, Janice. *Hard Knocks: Domestic Violence and the Psychology of Storytelling.* New York: Routledge, 2010.

Harrison, Kathryn. *The Kiss.* New York: Random House, 1997.

Heilbrun, Carolyn G. *Writing a Woman's Life.* New York: Ballantine Books, 1988.

Herman, Judith. *Trauma and Recovery: The Aftermath of Violence—from Domestic Abuse to Political Terror.* New York: Basic Books, 1992.

Bibliography

Higgins, Lynn A., and Brenda R. Silver, eds. *Rape and Representation.* New York: Columbia University Press, 1991.

Imarisha, Walidah, ed. *Octavia's Brood: Science Fiction Stories from Social Justice Movements.* Oakland, CA: AK Press, 2015.

International Association for Near-Death Experiences. "NDE Accounts." https://iands.org/research0/ndes/nde-stories/iands-nde -accounts.html.

Jayne, Bryan, and Joseph Buckley. *A Field Guide to the Reid Technique.* Chicago: Reid, 2015.

——. *The Investigator Anthology: A Compilation of Articles and Essays About the Reid Technique of Interviewing and Interrogation,* 2nd ed. Chicago: Reid, 2018.

Kalsched, Donald. *Trauma and the Soul: A Psycho-Spiritual Approach to Human Development and Its Interruption.* London: Routledge, 2013.

Lansbury, Coral. *The Old Brown Dog: Women, Workers, and Vivisection in Edwardian England.* Madison: University of Wisconsin Press, 1985.

Lonsway, Kimberly, and Jim Hopper. *Statement on Trauma-Informed Responses to Sexual Assault.* End Violence Against Women International, 2019.

Luke, Helen M. *Dark Wood to White Rose: Journey and Transformation in Dante's* Divine Comedy. New York: Parabola Books, 1989.

Miller, Julie B. "Eroticized Violence in Medieval Women's Mystical Literature: A Call for a Feminist Critique." *Journal of Feminist Studies in Religion* 15, no. 2 (Fall 1999): 25–49.

Olsen, Tillie. *Silences.* London: Virago, 1980.

Patterson, Debra. "The Impact of Detectives' Manner of Questioning on Rape Victims' Disclosure." *Violence Against Women* 17, no. 11 (2011): 1349–73.

Rauch, S. L., et al. "A Symptom Provocation Study of Posttraumatic Stress Disorder Using Positron Emission Tomography and Script-Driven Imagery." *Archives of General Psychiatry* 53, no. 5 (1996): 380–87.

Reid, John E. & Associates. *The Reid Technique of Interviewing and Interrogation: Special Edition (Course Handbook).* Chicago: Reid, 2000.

Rich, Adrienne. "When We Dead Awaken: Writing as Re-Vision." *College English* 34, no. 1, Women, Writing and Teaching (1972): 18–30.

Bibliography

Robinson, *Missy. Fierce & Fabulous.* Self-published.

Schwartz, Mark F., Lori D. Galperin, and William H. Masters. "Dissociation and Treatment of Compulsive Reenactment of Trauma: Sexual Compulsivity." In *Adult Survivors of Sexual Abuse: Treatment Innovations,* edited by Mic Hunter, 42–52. Thousand Oaks, CA: Sage Publications, 1995.

Serdahely, William J. "Near-Death Experiences and Dissociation: Two Cases." *Journal of Near-Death Studies* 12, no. 2 (Winter 1993): 85–94.

Singer, Margot, and Nicole Walker, eds. *Bending Genre: Essays on Creative Nonfiction.* New York: Bloomsbury, 2023.

Tatar, Maria. *Enchanted Hunters: The Power of Stories in Childhood.* New York: W. W. Norton, 2009.

——. *The Heroine with 1001 Faces.* Cambridge, MA: Harvard University Press, 2021.

Tylim, Isaac. "Imagining the Truth. Discussion of Prince's 'The Self in Pain: The Paradox of Memory. The Paradox of Testimony.'" *American Journal of Psychoanalysis* 69 (2009): 304–10.

Wilkinson, James John Garth. *The Forcible Introspection of Women for the Army and Navy by the Oligarchy, Considered Physically.* London: F. Pitman, 1870, 23–4.

Wise, Jessica. "Subaltern Women, Sexual Violence, and Trauma in Ovid's *Amores.*" In *Emotional Trauma in Greece and Rome: Representations and Reactions,* edited by Andromache Karanika and Vassiliki Panoussi, 71–92. London: Routledge, 2020.

Wisnicki, Adrian S., dir. *Livingstone's 1871 Field Diary.* Updated ed. In *Livingstone Online.* Adrian S. Wisnicki and Megan Ward, dirs. University of Maryland Libraries, 2017. http://livingstoneonline .org/uuid/node/75c25c6c-c491-4059-b446-3562d7518c95.

Fear and Trembling

Augusto Maieron, Mario. "The Meaning of Madness in Ancient Greek Culture from Homer to Hippocrates and Plato." *Medicina Historica* 1 (2017): 65–76.

Berceli, David. *The Revolutionary Trauma Release Process.* Vancouver: Namaste, 2008.

Bourguignon, Erika. "Suffering and Healing, Subordination and Power:

Women and Possession Trance." *Ethos* 32, no. 4 (December 2004): 557–74.

Cahun, Claude, Djuna Barnes, and Sharla Hutchison. "Convulsive Beauty: Images of Hysteria and Transgressive Sexuality." *Symploke* 11, no. 1–2 (2003): 212–26.

Devinsky, Orrin. "Nonepileptic Psychogenic Seizures: Quagmires of Pathophysiology, Diagnosis, and Treatment." *Epilepsia* 39 (1998): 458–62.

Faber, Diana P. "Jean-Martin Charcot and the Epilepsy/Hysteria Relationship." *Journal of the History of the Neurosciences* 6, no. 3 (1997): 275–90.

Gamgree, Arthur. "An Account of a Demonstration on the Phenomena of Hystero-Epilepsy Given by Professor Charcot at the Salpêtrière." October 12, 1878.

Goetz, G. "The Salpêtrière in the Wake of Charcot's Death." *Archives of Neurology* 44, no. 4 (1988): 444–47.

Harris, Grace. "Possession 'Hysteria' in a Kenya Tribe." *American Anthropologist* 59, no. 6 (December 1957): 1046–66.

Hecker, J. F. C. *The Black Death and the Dancing Mania.* Translated by B. G. Babington. London: Cassell & Company, 1888.

Hoff, Ann. "'I Was Convulsed, Pitiably Hideous': Convulsive Shock Treatment in Leonora Carrington's 'Down Below.'" *Journal of Modern Literature* 32, no. 3 (Spring 2009): 55–70.

Hustvedt, Asti. *Medical Muses: Hysteria in Nineteenth-Century Paris.* New York: W. W. Norton, 2011.

International League Against Epilepsy. "The History and Stigma of Epilepsy." *Epilepsia* 44, no. S6 (2003): 12–14.

Kraemer, Ross S. "Ecstasy and Possession: The Attraction of Women to the Cult of Dionysus." *Harvard Theological Review* 72, nos. 1–2 (January–April 1979): 55–80.

Magiorkinis, Emmanouil, Kalliopi Sidiropoulou, and Aristidis Diamantis. "Hallmarks in the History of Epilepsy: Epilepsy in Antiquity." *Epilepsy & Behavior* 5 (December 2009): 34–48.

Mappen, Marc. *Witches and Historians: Interpretations of Salem.* Malabar, FL: Robert Krieger Publishing, 1980.

Marshall, J. W. "Traumatic Dances of the Non-Self: Bodily Incoherence and the Hysterical Archive." In *Performing Hysteria: Images and Imaginations of Hysteria*, edited by J. Braun, 61–86. Belgium: Leuven University Press, 2020.

Myers, Lorna. *Psychogenic Nonepileptic Seizures: A Guide.* Self-published, 2014.

Oto, M., P. Conway, A. McGonigal, A. J. Russell, and R. Duncan. "Gender Differences in Psychogenic Non-Epileptic Seizures." *Seizure* 14, no. 1 (January 2005): 33–39.

Temkin, Owsei. *The Falling Sickness: A History of Epilepsy from the Greeks to the Beginnings of Modern Neurology.* Baltimore: Johns Hopkins Press, 1945.

Persephone, or To Bring Destruction

Deliramich, Aimee N., and Matt J. Gray. *Changes in Women's Sexual Behavior Following Sexual Assault.* Laramie: University of Wyoming Press, 2008.

Ernaux, Annie. *A Girl's Story.* Translated by Alison L. Strayer. New York: Seven Stories Press, 2020.

Glück, Louise. *Averno: Poems.* New York: Farrar, Straus and Giroux, 2007.

O'Callaghan, Erin, and Katherine Lorenz. " 'I Think I Just Like Having Sex': A Qualitative Study of Sexual Assault Survivors and Their Sexual Pleasure." *Sex Roles* 90 (2024): 1169–87.

I Really Think I Love You

Allison, Dorothy. *Bastard out of Carolina.* New York: Plume, 1992.

Constantine, David. *In Another Country.* Biblioasis, 2015.

Critelli, Joseph W., and Jenny M. Bivona. "Women's Erotic Rape Fantasies: An Evaluation of Theory and Research." *Journal of Sex Research* 45, no. 1 (2008): 57–70.

Ford, Jessie. " 'Going with the Flow': How College Men's Experiences of Unwanted Sex Are Produced by Gendered Interactional Pressures." *Social Forces* 96, no. 3 (March 2018): 1303–24.

———. "Unwanted Sex on Campus: The Overlooked Role of Interactional Pressures and Gendered Sexual Scripts." *Qualitative Sociology* 44 (2021): 31–53.

Ford, Jessie, and Andréa Becker. " 'A Situation Where There Aren't Rules': Unwanted Sex for Gay, Bisexual, and Questioning Men." *Sociological Science* 7 (2020): 57–74.

Bibliography

Ford, Jessie, and Christopher Maggio. "How College Men Understand Unwanted Sex with Women." *Sociological Forum* 35 (2020): 648–72.

Ford, Jessie, Aarushi Shah, Gloria Fortuna, and Jennifer Hirsch. "Embodied Injustice: Comparing Lesbian, Bisexual, and Queer and Heterosexual Women's Accounts of Unwanted Sex." *Social Currents* 1 (2024): 1–17.

Kennelly, Brian G. "Rape Fantasy Redux? Textual Victimhood in and Between Versions of Tony Duvert's *Portrait d'homme couteau*." *Dalhousie French Studies* 101 (2014): 93–103.

Peele, Stanton, and Archie Brodsky. *Love and Addiction.* New York: Signet, 2015.

Schaeffer, Brenda. *Is It Love or Is It Addiction: The Book That Changed the Way We Think About Romance and Intimacy.* Illustrated edition. Center City, MN: Hazelden Publishing, 2009.

West, Robin. "Consensual Sexual Dysphoria: A Challenge for Campus Life." *Journal of Legal Education* 66, no. 4 (2017): 804–21.

Another Sleeping Beauty

Nussbaum, Martha. "Beyond Obsession and Disgust: Lucretius' Genealogy of Love Werner." *Apeiron* 22, no. 1 (1989): 1–60.

One Day at a Women's Prison

Chen, Xiaojin, et al. "Early Sexual Abuse, Street Adversity, and Drug Use Among Female Homeless and Runaway Adolescents in the Midwest." *Journal of Drug Issues* 34, no. 1 (2004): 1–21.

Chicago Torture Justice Center. "The Survivor Repair Fund." https://www.chicagotorturejustice.org/repairfund.

Dobash, R. Emerson, et al. "Lethal and Nonlethal Violence Against an Intimate Female Partner: Comparing Male Murderers to Nonlethal Abusers." *Violence Against Women* (2007): 329, 345.

Illinois Executive Clemency Petition for Antheshia Lee, submitted by Rachel White-Domain, Attorney, Illinois Prison Project: July 22, 2021.

Illinois Executive Clemency Petition for Debraca Harris, submitted by Rachel White-Domain, Attorney, Illinois Prison Project: December 18, 2020.

Bibliography

Illinois Executive Clemency Petition for Laconda McDonald, submitted by Rachel White-Domain, Attorney, Illinois Prison Project: June 8, 2001.

Paine, M. L., and D. Hansen. "Factors Influencing Children to Self-Disclose Sexual Abuse." *Clinical Psychology Review* (2002): 271.

Pittman, Jacqueline. "Constructing Race and Gender in Modern Rape Law: The Abandoned Category of Black Female Victims." *Michigan Journal of Gender & Law* 30 (2023): 151.

Thacker, Lily Katherine, "The Danger of 'No': Rejection Violence, Toxic Masculinity and Violence Against Women." *Eastern Kentucky University* (2019).

Vera-Gray, Fiona. *Men's Intrusion, Women's Embodiment: A Critical Analysis of Street Harassment.* New York: Routledge, 2017.

No, No, No

Dorr, Lisa Lindquist. *White Women, Rape, and the Power of Race in Virginia, 1900–1960.* Chapel Hill: University of North Carolina Press, 2004.

Giddings, Paula. *Where and When I Enter: The Impact of Black Women on Race and Sex in America.* New York: William Morrow, 1984.

Hodes, Martha. "The Sexualization of Reconstruction Politics: White Women and Black Men in the South After the Civil War." *Journal of the History of Sexuality* 3, no. 3 (1993): 402–17.

Martenzie, Johnson. "Being Black in a World Where White Lies Matter." *Andscape*, January 30, 2017.

Natanson, Hannah. "When Black Lives Matter Came to White Rural America." *The Washington Post*, July 27, 2020.

Tal, Kalí. *Worlds of Hurt: Reading the Literatures of Trauma.* New York: Cambridge University Press, 1996.

Luisa's Escape

Hinton, Devon, and Bryon J. Good, eds. *Culture and PTSD: Trauma in Global and Historical Perspective.* Philadelphia: University of Pennsylvania Press, 2016.

LaCapra, Dominick. *Writing History, Writing Trauma.* Baltimore: Johns Hopkins University Press, 2001.

Bibliography

Rajiva, Jay. *Postcolonial Parabola: Literature, Tactility, and the Ethics of Representing Trauma*. London: Bloomsbury, 2017.

Rothberg, Michael. "Decolonizing Trauma Studies: A Response." *Studies in the Novel* 40, nos. 1–2 (Spring & Summer 2008): 224–34.

Schneider, Luisa T. *Love and Violence in Sierra Leone: Mediating Intimacy After Conflict*. Cambridge: Cambridge University Press, 2025.

———. "Rape, Ritual, Rupture, and Repair: Decentering Euro-American Logics of Trauma and Healing in an Analytic Autoethnography of the Five Years After My Rape in Sierra Leone." *Ethos* 51, no. 3 (September 2023): 255–70.

———. "Sexual Violence During Research: How the Unpredictability of Fieldwork and the Right to Risk Collide with Academic Bureaucracy and Expectations." *Critique of Anthropology* 40, no. 2 (2020): 173–93.

JEN PERCY is a contributing writer at *The New York Times Magazine* and recipient of the National Magazine Award for Feature Writing. She is also the author of *Demon Camp*, a *New York Times* Notable Book. Percy has received numerous awards, including a Pushcart Prize, a Dart Award for Excellence in Coverage of Trauma, a National Endowment for the Arts grant, and fellowships from the Bread Loaf Writers' Conference and MacDowell. A graduate of the University of Iowa's Nonfiction Writing Program and the Iowa Writers' Workshop, Percy's work has appeared in *The New York Times Book Review, Harper's Magazine, The New Republic, Esquire,* and elsewhere. She teaches writing at New York University's Arthur L. Carter Journalism Institute.

A Note on the Type

This book was set in Amiri, a classical Arabic typeface designed in the Naskh style—a small, round script of Islamic calligraphy. It was designed and digitized in 2017 by Khaled Hosny as a revival of the 1905 typeface used by the Bulaq Press (also known as the Amiriya Press, from where the font gets its name). Though designed with setting Arabic type in mind, the Roman version is elegant and highly readable, making it suitable for setting books and running text.

Typeset by Scribe, Philadelphia, Pennsylvania

Book designed by Betty Lew

01 14
J